PHARMA
KINETICS, AN
PERSONALIZED MEDICINE

David F. Kisor, BS, PharmD, RPh

Professor of Pharmacokinetics
Chair, Department of Pharmaceutical and Biomedical Sciences
Ohio Northern University
The Raabe College of Pharmacy
Ada, Ohio

Michael D. Kane, PhD

Associate Professor of Bioinformatics and Genomics
Department of Computer and Information Technology
College of Technology
Purdue University
West Lafayette, Indiana

Jeffery N. Talbot, PhD

Associate Professor of Pharmacology
Department of Pharmaceutical and Biomedical Sciences
Ohio Northern University
The Raabe College of Pharmacy
Ada, Ohio

Jon E. Sprague, PhD, RPh

Professor of Pharmacology
Dean, Raabe College of Pharmacy
Ohio Northern University
The Raabe College of Pharmacy
Ada, Ohio

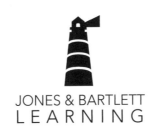

JONES & BARTLETT
L E A R N I N G

World Headquarters
Jones & Bartlett Learning
5 Wall Street
Burlington, MA 01803
978-443-5000
info@jblearning.com
www.jblearning.com

Jones & Bartlett's books and products are available through most bookstores and online booksellers. To contact Jones & Bartlett Learning directly, call 800-832-0034, fax 978-443-8000, or visit our website, www.jblearning.com.

Production Credits
Publisher: William Brottmiller
Senior Acquisitions Editor: Katey Birtcher
Editorial Assistant: Kayla Dos Santos
Editorial Assistant: Sean Fabery
Production Editor: Jessica Steele Newfell
Marketing Manager: Grace Richards
Manufacturing and Inventory Control Supervisor: Amy Bacus
Composition: Laserwords Private Limited, Chennai, India
Cover Design: Michael O'Donnell
Cover Images: (DNA strand) © Photodisc; (pills) © Photos.com
Title Page Image: (pills) © Photos.com
Printing and Binding: Edwards Brothers Malloy
Cover Printing: Edwards Brothers Malloy

To order this product, use ISBN: 978-1-4496-5273-9

Library of Congress Cataloging-in-Publication Data
Pharmacogenetics, kinetics, and dynamics for personalized medicine / by David F. Kisor ... [et al.].
    p. ; cm.
Includes bibliographical references and index.
ISBN 978-1-4496-3393-6 — ISBN 1-4496-3393-5
I. Kisor, David F.
[DNLM: 1. Pharmacogenetics. 2. Individualized Medicine. 3. Pharmacokinetics. QV 38.5]
    615.7—dc23
                                                                    2012041082
6048

Printed in the United States of America
17 16 15 14 13   10 9 8 7 6 5 4 3 2 1

Contents

Preface

This initial offering of *Pharmacogenetics, Kinetics, and Dynamics for Personalized Medicine* is intended as a "foundation" text for pharmacy students. The work is not a comprehensive reference source. Rather, the text is written to help the student develop a solid knowledge base that interfaces the "newer" discipline of pharmacogenetics with our understanding of the more established disciplines of pharmacokinetics and pharmacodynamics. The foundations presented will serve as a basis for understanding some of the observed variability seen in pharmacokinetics and pharmacodynamics among various populations of patients and in the individual patient.

In Section I of this text, the authors have described the basic mechanisms of the expression of genetic information and the variation expressed in the genotype and phenotype of individuals. This section describes how genetic variation can explain an individual's response to drug therapy. This section is written in a narrative style to "tell a story" that encompasses the broad topic of genetics and the application of genetics and drugs (i.e., pharmacogenetics and pharmacogenomics) to patient care.

Section II of this text focuses on the relationships between pharmacogenetics and how the body handles a drug (pharmacokinetics) and pharmacogenetics and how a drug affects the body (pharmacodynamics). Here, the genetic basis for altered drug absorption, distribution, metabolism, excretion, and drug action is presented, with numerous "genetic–kinetic interfaces" and "genetic–dynamic interfaces." As the student will be presented with mathematical equations in the framework of pharmacokinetics and pharmacodynamics, this section describes how pharmacokinetic and pharmacodynamic parameters are influenced by an individual's genetic constitution, leading to the need for an altered dose or, in some cases, alternative drug therapy. Example equations are provided to show how genetics plays a role in dosage design and calculation from a mathematical standpoint. Numerous examples are provided in structured tables and figures, and key terms and key equations are provided as well.

With respect to the key terms, some terms lack consistent definitions, as various authors and organizations define the same term differently. For instance, we utilize the brief definitions of pharmacogenetics and pharmacogenomics found on the Pharmacogenomics Knowledge Base website, and we utilize the abbreviations for these terms, PGt and PGx, respectively, as provided by the U.S. Food and Drug Administration (FDA). Although authors may have their own definitions for these terms, we have decided to utilize those from an established source so as to not introduce further confusion. Regardless, a glossary is provided with definitions of terms used in this text. While it would be optimal to have consistent definitions and abbreviations, the use of different definitions and abbreviations across the literature should be viewed as an opportunity to question oneself and think about a term from different points of view.

Section III presents a number of specific drugs, describing relationships between genetics and drug action and how the body handles the particular drug. We look at specific examples of genetics related to adverse drug reactions, altered metabolism, and drug efficacy. In each chapter in this section, learning objectives include case questions that are answered at the end of each chapter. As in Section II, genetic–kinetic and genetic–dynamic interfaces are presented. At the time of publishing this first edition, there are approximately 33 oncology drugs and 27 psychiatry drugs that have genomic information in their package labels. We chose not to provide a chapter on each of these drugs. Instead, we chose to provide "example" drug chapters from across a multitude of therapeutic areas that provide a foundation for understanding pharmacogenetics. Certainly we will add more drug chapters, either as online supplements and/or as chapters in future editions.

For the science of pharmacogenetics to be applied clinically, many issues beyond the interface of genetics with kinetics and dynamics must be considered. In Section IV, we have chosen to briefly discuss a number of these issues and present the information as introductory material because volumes can and have been written about each topic. This section includes introductory information on the cost of sequencing a whole genome, education in pharmacogenetics, genetic privacy, and pharmacogenomics resources, among other topics.

We believe that personalized medicine is in its infancy and that a key component in advancing personalized medicine to an accepted standard of care is the education of pharmacy students. Although there are many hurdles to the implementation of personalized medicine, education is the key to overcoming these hurdles.

In the future, it is likely that an individual's genome will be sequenced early in life, likely with a DNA sample obtained at birth. For the most part, individual genetic testing will no longer be required because the whole-genome information, stored in a secure database, will be available for query when an "actionable" intervention can be made to optimize drug therapy. We truly hope that this work provides a basis for the understanding of pharmacogenetics relative to personalized medicine, thus expanding the role of the pharmacist to interpret and apply pharmacogenetic information to optimize drug therapy, serving the patients to the best of our abilities.

Acknowledgments

The authors are indebted to numerous individuals who have helped review and shape this effort. We would like to thank all of our students for their inspiration and specifically those who served as initial reviewers of the material, including Michael E. Spiller, Olivia Hollot, Nicole E. Sivak, MaryAnne M. Ventura, Olivia Hiddleson, Shane M. Parks, Brian C. Thomas, Katherine M. Lorson, Joanne K. Tran, Adam Trimble, Lauren Desko, and Elizabeth M. Calcei. Finally, we would like to thank the numerous external reviewers of this text. Their constructive input and comments helped "hone" specific chapters and improve this text overall.

About the Authors

David F. Kisor

Dr. Kisor is Professor and Chair of the Department of Pharmaceutical and Biomedical Sciences at the Raabe College of Pharmacy at Ohio Northern University. Kisor received his Bachelor of Science degree in Pharmacy from the University of Toledo and his PharmD from The Ohio State University. He completed a fellowship in Therapeutic Drug Monitoring and Pharmacokinetics at Ohio State. Kisor came to ONU from Burroughs Wellcome Co., now GlaxoSmithKline, where he was a research scientist in Pharmacokinetics and Drug Metabolism, working mostly on the development of purine analogs, including the drug nelarabine, a derivative of guanine, one of the "building blocks of life," that was marketed in the United States in 2005. His focus at ONU has been teaching pharmacokinetics and relating genetics to pharmacokinetics. He has integrated pharmacogenetics into the pharmacokinetic subject matter since 1998. He is a member of the American Pharmacists Association (APhA), the American Association of Colleges of Pharmacy (AACP), the National Coalition for Health Professional

Education in Genetics (NCHPEG), and the Personalized Medicine Coalition (PMC) and is the advisor for the ONU Student Chapter of the PMC.

Michael D. Kane

Dr. Kane's professional experience includes performing preclinical research in the pharmaceutical industry, serving as Vice President of Research and Development at a publicly traded genomics/biotechnology company, and cofounding several companies based on technology and methods that he has developed and patented. His primary interests have involved the development and utilization of genomic-detection technologies, primarily DNA microarray methods, which have been applied to exploratory discovery efforts in agriculture, ecology, and preclinical and clinical studies. In addition, he has led efforts to develop data management tools in support of pharmacogenomics and personalized medicine, which have been extensively utilized as a teaching tool for healthcare professionals. Dr. Kane also serves as an expert witness in criminal cases involving DNA evidence. His hobbies include custom conversions of electric vehicles as well as building and playing custom electric guitars.

Jeffery N. Talbot

Dr. Talbot received a BS degree in Biochemistry from the University of Nevada. He went on to earn a PhD in Pharmacology from the University of Nebraska Medical Center, utilizing yeast genetics to identify and characterize novel regulators of G protein-coupled receptors in the central nervous system. Talbot continued his studies as a National Institute on Drug Abuse (NIDA) research fellow at the University of Michigan Medical School, where he investigated the effects of transgene-mediated mutations on neurotransmitter function in mouse genetic models. At the Raabe College of Pharmacy at Ohio Northern University, Talbot teaches fourth- and fifth-year pharmacy students on topics including neuronal communications, drug action in the central nervous system, and genetic influence on drug responses. He also directs preclinical research utilizing genetically modified mice to explore novel treatments for drug abuse and depression.

Jon E. Sprague

Dr. Sprague is a Professor of Pharmacology and Dean at the Raabe College of Pharmacy at Ohio Northern University. Before returning to ONU as Dean in 2006, Dr. Sprague was Professor and Chair of Pharmacology at the Virginia College of Osteopathic Medicine at Virginia Tech University. He received his PhD in Pharmacology and Toxicology from Purdue University and his Pharmacy degree from Ferris State University. His research interests include studying the hyperthermic mechanisms of the substituted amphetamines, namely 3,4-methylene-dioxy-methamphetamine (i.e., MDMA, Ecstasy). One of Dr. Sprague's major professional priorities is to assist in the implementation of personalized medicine to improve health outcomes.

© Mauro Saivezzo/ShutterStock, Inc.

Reviewers

Mahfoud Assem, PharmD, PhD
Assistant Professor, College of Pharmacy
University of Iowa
Iowa City, Iowa

Ganesh Cherala, PhD
Assistant Professor, College of Pharmacy
Oregon State University
Portland, Oregon

R. Stephanie Huang, PhD
Assistant Professor, Department of Medicine
University of Chicago
Chicago, Illinois

J. Shawn Jones, PhD, MS
Assistant Professor, School of Pharmacy
University of Charleston
Charleston, West Virginia

Craig A.H. Richard, PhD
Associate Professor, School of Pharmacy
Shenandoah University
Winchester, Virginia

Venkataramana Vooradi, PhD, RPh
Pharmacist
Apothecary Drugs, Inc.
Okemos, Michigan

Additional feedback was considered from reviewers who wished to remain anonymous.

Pharmacogenetics, Kinetics, and Dynamics for Personalized Medicine

Section I presents, in a narrative manner, genetics related to evolution. The structure of the genome and its regulation are discussed in terms of the underlying cell biology. Variations in the genome are connected to personalized medicine, describing specific types of polymorphisms and their relationship to phenotypes and drug response.

Chapter 1

Introduction to Personalized Medicine

LEARNING OBJECTIVES

Upon completion of this chapter, the student will be able to:

1. Recognize basic mechanisms of the expression of genetic information as traits—from the deoxyribonucleic acid (DNA) sequence to transcribed ribonucleic acid (RNA), to translated proteins, to phenotype.
2. Differentiate among the major types of genetic variation, including non-synonymous, synonymous, nonsense single nucleotide polymorphisms (SNPs), and insertion/deletion (indel) polymorphisms in both genotypic and phenotypic terms.
3. Provide specific examples that establish the relationship between altered drug disposition and polymorphic cytochrome P450 enzymes.
4. Describe how polymorphic genetic variation can be utilized to predict individualized responses to drug therapy.

Key Terms	Definition
allele	Alternate sequences or versions of the same gene inherited from each parent.
biomarker (genomic)	A measurable DNA and/or RNA characteristic that is an indicator of normal biologic processes, pathogenic processes, and/or response to therapeutic or other interventions.
codon	Three adjacent nucleotide bases that ultimately encodes a specific amino acid.
exon	A nucleotide sequence that codes information for protein synthesis.
gene	Regions of the genome (DNA) that contain the instructions to make proteins.
genome	The entire DNA of an organism.
genotype	The specific set of alleles inherited at a locus on a given gene.
haplotype	A series of polymorphisms that are inherited together.
heterozygous	Possessing two different alleles for the same trait.
histone	A protein around which DNA coils to form chromatin, thus "packaging" DNA.
homozygous	Possessing identical alleles for the same trait.
indel	Insertion or deletion of DNA either as single nucleotides or spanning regions of DNA involving many nucleotides.
intron	A nucleotide sequence in DNA that does not code information for protein synthesis and is removed before translation of messenger RNA.
monogenic trait	Characteristics derived from a single gene.
multigenic trait	Characteristics derived from multiple genes.
mutation	A change in DNA sequence between individuals.
nucleotide	One of the structural components, or building blocks, of DNA, including adenine (A), cytosine (C), guanine (G), and thymine (T), and of RNA, including adenine (A), cytosine (C), guanine (G), and uracil (U).
personalized medicine	The use of patient-specific information and biomarkers to make more informed choices regarding the optimal therapeutic treatment regimen for a given patient.
pharmacodynamics (PD)	The relationship between drug exposure and pharmacologic response.
pharmacogenetics (PGt)	The study of a gene involved in response to a drug.
pharmacogenomics (PGx)	The study of many genes, in some cases the entire genome, involved in response to a drug.
pharmacokinetics (PK)	The relationship of time and drug absorption, distribution, metabolism, and excretion.
phenotype	An individual's expression of a physical trait or physiologic function due to genetic makeup and environmental and other factors.
polymorphism	A mutation in DNA in a given population that may be observed at greater than 1% frequency.
reference sequence number (refSNP, rs#, rs)	A unique and consistent identifier of a given single nucleotide polymorphism (SNP).
single nucleotide polymorphism (SNP)	A variant DNA sequence in which a single nucleotide has been replaced by another base.
topoisomerase	A class of enzymes that alter the supercoiling of double-stranded DNA.
wild-type	The typical or normally occurring genotype of an organism.
xenobiotics	Substances (often drugs) introduced into the body but not produced by it.

Introduction

In its simplest terms, **personalized medicine** is the use of patient-specific information and **biomarkers** to make more informed choices regarding the optimal therapeutic treatment regimen for that patient, rather than reliance on population-based therapeutic trends. **Pharmacogenetics (PGt)** is the aspect of personalized medicine whereby patient-specific genomic biomarkers are used to choose the optimal drug and/or dose for the patient, with the goal of assuring drug efficacy in the patient while minimizing or avoiding the risk of an adverse drug reaction. The successful implementation of pharmacogenetics in the clinic is dependent upon a number of different processes and data, including *a priori* knowledge about a specific **allele** in the genome and its linkage to altered **pharmacokinetics (PK)** and/or **pharmacodynamics (PD)** (compared to the statistical norm in the population), the ability to accurately test a patient for the presence of a specific allele in his or her genome, and the ability to offer the patient more effective alternatives than would be typically offered to a patient in the statistical norm of the population. Key to this process is the utilization of prior discoveries and clinical findings (e.g., data) regarding a specific genomic allele relevant to the pharmacokinetics and/or pharmacodynamics of the prescribed or intended drug, and then *predicting* how the patient will respond to the drug. Finally, the utilization of pharmacogenetics and personalized medicine must add value to healthcare. In other words, the costs associated with the implementation and utilization of pharmacogenetics and personalized medicine must be ethically and economically justified by reducing the negative (adverse) effects and costs associated with adverse drug reactions as well as the assurance of more effective drug therapy outcomes for the healthcare consumer population.

Here, we distinguish the term *pharmacogenetics* from the now more commonly used **pharmacogenomics (PGx)**. In its purest sense, pharmacogenetics refers to the study of a gene involved in response to a drug, whereas pharmacogenomics (PGx) refers to the study of all genes in the genome involved in response to a drug.[1] However, the vernacular that has emerged in recent years often uses the term *pharmacogenomics* to reference the entirety of the science and the methods that study the interface of genomics, genetics, and drugs used in clinical therapeutics.

Living Systems and the Genome

The adult human body contains trillions of different cells, each performing different functions to sustain life. Some of these are muscle cells, some make up our skin, some are blood cells, some form bone, some are brain or liver cells, and so on. Each of these cells has developed within a specific tissue in the body to perform a specific function. For example, our red blood cells are capable of transporting molecular oxygen from our lungs to organs and tissues, and then transporting carbon dioxide back to the lungs to be removed from the body. This unique cellular capability is due to the presence of a specific protein in the red blood cell called hemoglobin. More specifically, what we commonly refer to as hemoglobin is actually a multimolecular structure that contains a heterocyclic organic molecule called heme, which is bound to an atom of iron, as well as two specific globular proteins. These globular proteins are alpha-globulin and beta-globulin, which are each derived from a specific gene in our genome. Thus, the genes are used by the cellular machinery as a "blueprint" or "instruction set" on how to make these proteins. Hence, **genes** are the regions of our genome that contain the instructions to make proteins, and proteins are the functional components of living systems. In simpler terms, if the genes are the "blueprints" for life, then proteins are the "bricks and mortar" of living systems. Proteins are the inherited, functional components of living organisms—inherited because they are derived from our genome, which we inherit from our parents and ancestors. Interestingly, less than 2% of our genome is actually used as template genes to make proteins.[2] We will discuss aspects of proteins later; let us first take a closer look at our genome.

The **genome** of an organism is the instruction set for that organism, or, more specifically, the instruction set for the development of its cells and tissues, as well as the maintenance of these cells and tissues throughout the life of the organism. The functional molecule that makes up our genome is DNA (deoxyribonucleic acid). Our genome is made up of four different DNA **nucleotide** bases (adenine-A, cytosine-C, guanine-G, and thymine-T), which are somewhat equivalent to a written language with four different letters. The human genome contains about three billion nucleotide bases (or letters; A, C, G, T) in the genome, and essentially each cell (that contains a nucleus) contains a copy of the entire genome. To appreciate the size of the human genome, consider that, if our genome was printed in paperback novel form, it would contain over four million pages. By no means is the human genome considered large within the spectrum of living organisms on earth. The onion (yes, the one you eat) has a genome that is more than six times the size of the human genome, and it has been estimated that certain lilies (flowering plants) have a genome that is 30 times bigger than our own.[3,4] We will not be discussing the complexities of plant genomes in this textbook, as scientists are only beginning to understand the different complex genomes in living organisms.

If we take the perspective of our genome representing information, then we must recognize that each cell has the instructions (genes) for all the proteins that the organism can ever make, even though the cell may not use all this information. In other words, each cell (that has a nucleus) has all of the chromosomes of the genome, and therefore all the genes that we have inherited from our parents, yet each cell only uses a subset of these genes to make the proteins it needs to thrive and carry out its various functions. To conceptualize this phenomenon, imagine that each person in your college or organization was a cell, and each person has a computer that contains all the programs needed to make the entire organization run successfully. A person working in the accounting office would use the computer programs (i.e., genes) that are used to manage the organization's resources and inventory but would not use the programs used for personnel management (even though those programs are stored on the computer). Similarly, a muscle cell uses the genes to make the proteins used for mechanical contraction, but not the genes that make the proteins for detecting light that are used in the retinal cells of the eye.

Genetic Evolution and the Evolution of Genetics

Sexual reproduction is the fundamental process for enabling genetic diversity and the propagation of life on earth. It involves the passing of genetic information from viable parent organisms to their offspring. Thus, the offspring inherit the genetic information that allowed their parent organisms to thrive and survive in the environment. Furthermore, it allows two different successful organisms (the biological mother and father) with different genomic content to create variations of their respective genomes in their offspring, thereby creating genetically varied offspring. The life of these offspring represents a test of the content of their genome, and reaching sexual maturity and successfully reproducing reinforces the rigor of their genomic content (i.e., the viability of the organism was sufficient to endure its environment), which is passed on to subsequent generations. This is the basis of natural selection, or "survival of the fittest," from the perspective of the inherited genome. The genetic variability among the population (of a given species) appears extremely important for the evolutionary success of the species because it allows the species to adapt to changes in its environment over generations by reinforcing the traits that confer viability. In other words, as changes in the environment emerge and exert selective pressure on the species, members of the population that harbor the genetic content (that encode physical or behavioral traits) to overcome these environmental changes survive and shape the genetic content and physical traits of subsequent generations. This process is a fundamental tenet of evolution on earth.

We are all familiar with the genetic diversity and variation in the human population, as evidenced by obvious physical traits, such as eye color, hair color, and so on. These physical traits are the result of inherited genes from our biological parents, and dictate aspects of our physical appearance. This genetic variation extends into many aspects of our genome and cell biology that are not always as obvious, such as those that affect behavior or aspects of cellular biology. These variations in the human population are very important to the perpetuation of our species. As our regional and planetary environments change over long periods of time, those individuals that are best suited to survive in the changing environment will thrive and continue to bear offspring. The makeup of our genome, and therefore our physiology, is the result of millions of years of evolution under the selective pressures of our environment as well as competition for survival. In other words, the physical and behavioral traits that provided our ancestors with a competitive advantage allowed those individuals to thrive and bear offspring, whereas individuals who lacked a given competitive advantage were much less likely to thrive and bear offspring. Therefore, the individuals that harbored advantageous traits passed their genes onto their offspring, and after thousands of generations of human evolution the content of our genome is the result of this evolutionary process. Thus, our genome contains the genes that conferred the beneficial traits needed for our ancestors to thrive.

These traits may be very subtle yet important, such as the ability to digest lactose into adulthood and therefore derive sustenance from the milk of the beasts of burden that our ancestors domesticated over the last 10,000 years. Our ancestors who experienced this evolutionary adaptation could better survive periods of famine and drought, and this trait was retained in our recent evolution. It should become obvious that the changes in our genetic makeup that resulted in specific competitive advantages would be passed down through generations, whereas changes in our genome that did not serve a beneficial purpose, or in many cases even reduced the viability of an individual, are not seen in the modern human genome. Hence, we are the modern beneficiaries of this genetic "arms race" of inherited traits that has been ongoing for millions of years.

When we consider the past influences that have shaped our biology and the content of our genome, we can begin to understand why exposure to certain chemicals and compounds that we may ingest pose a threat to our survival whereas other substances are safe. For example, certain mushrooms (e.g., the death cap mushroom) and frogs (e.g., the poison dart frog of South America) synthesize compounds that are toxic to organisms that would otherwise consume them as a nutrient source. The death cap mushroom synthesizes a compound called amanitin, and the poisonous dart frog synthesizes epibatidine (among other alkaloids). It is well known that these compounds are highly toxic to humans and many other organisms.[5]

No evidence suggests that there are variations in the sensitivity to these poisons among humans, and thus we all avoid consuming these mushrooms and frogs, an adaptation that benefits the mushroom and the frog. Because these organisms, and their poisons, have existed in nature for millions of years alongside our ancestors, it is not necessary to consider variations in the toxicity of the poisonous compounds across the modern human population. Building upon our evolutionary theory, we can imagine a fictionalized paradigm of selective pressure 50,000 years ago where these mushrooms were abundant and only a subpopulation of humans harbored the ability to detoxify the poison in the mushroom and therefore safely consume the mushroom as a nutrient source. If this were the case and the mushrooms were an abundant source of nutrients, the humans that could safely consume the mushrooms would thrive, whereas the humans that were sensitive to the toxin would be less likely to thrive. In this fictitious example, it is likely that all humans living today would harbor the ability to detoxify and safely consume the poison simply due to selective pressure on our ancestors. In genomic terms, modern humans would harbor a gene in their genome that encoded an enzyme capable of breaking down the poison. Although this is not true for the poisons mentioned in this example, it is true for many other substances in nature that our ancestors encountered.

The example above is presented to demonstrate a fundamental difference between naturally occurring substances and modern pharmaceutical products. When we look at modern pharmaceutical compounds, we see a much more varied response among humans to both the safety and efficacy of these compounds, even though the process of drug development attempts to provide drugs that are efficacious and safe for the entire population. One reason for the varied responses to drugs is that these pharmaceutical compounds did *not* exist in nature and were not available for consumption by our ancestors. Therefore, no evolutionary selective pressures have been experienced in humans with respect to exposure to these pharmaceutical compounds, and the outcome of evolutionary selective pressure has not been manifested in the genome through thousands of generations. Thus, we expect a much more varied response in the population to these modern medicinal chemicals, compared to naturally occurring substances.

The development of safe and effective medicinal compounds is a challenge because there can be a spectrum of responses in the population regarding the safety and efficacy of a drug, and this can complicate the management of pharmacy and therapeutics in our modern healthcare system. In other words, due to the methods used to assess and approve new drug entities, modern drug approval requires that it be safe and effective in a large majority of the population. Thus, drugs under development that have shown large variation as to their safety and/or efficacy have not gained marketing approval. It should be obvious that if the genetic basis for variations within the population to the safety and/or efficacy of a drug are studied and understood, then a drug that is effective in a known subpopulation could be approved, if that subpopulation can be identified through genomic testing (i.e., pharmacogenetics or pharmacogenomics). In fact, this movement in pharmacotherapy will result in safer and more effective drug use within subpopulations in our society and enable healthcare professionals to use genomic screening to predict how a patient will respond to a specific drug and therefore inform healthcare professionals as to which drug and/or dose is optimal for the patient. This is a principal tenet for the adoption of personalized medicine.

We have discussed how selective pressure and evolution have shaped the content of our genome, now let us look at our genome from a completely different perspective: How have advances in modern healthcare and disease management or, more specifically, extending the length of human life, inadvertently revealed (or invented) a new type of genetic predisposition to disease?

At some time in our recent history, pre-modern humans lived together in groups composed primarily of three generations (i.e., children, parents, and grandparents). In a simple version of anthropological theory, the parental generation (in the physical prime of their life) worked to search for resources, gather food, and defend the group, while the elders helped oversee the young of the group. It is important to note that larger groups of individuals consume, and therefore require, more resources (e.g., food, water) than smaller groups. Thus, larger groups of early humans were at a disadvantage in times of limited resources (e.g., drought, famine), compared to smaller groups. Therefore, it was not beneficial for pre-modern humans to have a long lifespan, as this would result in large groups that were at a competitive disadvantage; for this reason human life expectancy was much shorter than it is today.

Australopithecines appear to have had an average life expectancy of only 15 to 20 years and survived for about 300,000 generations, ending about two million years ago. More recently, early agriculturalists and nomadic pre-modern humans had an average life span of about 25 years and survived only about 500 generations. These ancestral life spans suggest that age-related declines in function after the age of 25 were due to the forces of natural selection. In modern times, the last 200 years of human history (about 10 generations), the average life span has increased from 43 to 75 years of age.[6]

If we consider that the vast majority of our ancestors only had life expectancies of younger than 45 years, then certainly their genomic content and function was to maintain optimal health until this age, with no evolutionary advantage to extending life span. The increase in life expectancy between pre-modern and post-modern humans is nearly instantaneous as compared to the much longer timelines associated with pre-modern human evolution. For the purposes of illuminating this perspective, it can be assumed that our genome is essentially identical to our pre-modern ancestors' of 5,000 years ago.

In other words, the modern human genome has evolved to support an individual's life until they reach about 45 years old (this may even be a generous estimate), even if living in a modern society. Or, more accurately, any health problems that have a basis in genetics would not have been passed down from our ancestors if the health problem manifested itself early in life (i.e., before about 35 years). However, if the genetic-based health problem manifests itself after the age of 45 years, it would not have exerted selective pressure against individuals that harbored this genetic allele. Therefore, it would not have negatively impacted the survival of our pre-modern ancestors, and it would be expected to be present in our genome today. In other words, extending human life beyond the age of 50 years "reveals" new diseases in the human population, and the management of these age-related disorders becomes more dependent on modern healthcare methods, practices, and technology as we age. From this perspective, if it is determined that an individual has a genetic predisposition for a disease or disorder with an expected onset at 60 years of age, it is not a failure of human evolutionary processes but simply an artifact of extending human life.

Many examples of age-related disorders with genetic underpinnings can be found in humans, and it is certain that more discoveries will be made linking specific genetic markers with age-related disorders. An example of an age-related disorder with a known genetic link is Huntington's disease. Huntington's disease involves an inherited genetic defect where an expansion of a three nucleotide repeat (CAG) in the protein-coding region of a specific gene (named Huntington) causes the protein to self-aggregate. The deleterious effects (symptoms) of this genetic defect are usually first manifested at about 40 years of age. Thus, there were no selective pressures to eliminate this genetic defect from the population in pre-modern humans because it was not a genetic defect until our life expectancy increased beyond 40 years. This can be said for essentially all genetically linked diseases in humans older than 40 years of age.

As we consider age-related diseases, the ability to utilize genomic screening in the clinic is very important in identifying people who are predisposed to a specific age-dependent disorder. Ideally, utilizing genomic screening in this paradigm allows the patient ample time to take measures to reduce or eliminate the risk of the disorder, such as changes in diet, exercise, prophylactic medicines, and so on. In this case, it is important to note that although there is currently no "cure" for Huntington's disease, the disease can be diagnosed using genetic screening methods prior to the appearance of any disease symptoms. Thus, the use of genetic screening methods for disease risk should be carried out with adequate genetic counseling because (1) the results of genetic screening must be interpreted correctly and (2) there can be significant psychological ramifications associated with the results of genetic screening for the patient and family.

Genome Structure and Gene Regulation

Less than 2% of the human genome is made up of gene sequences that encode proteins, and these genes are distributed throughout the 23 chromosomes and mitochondrial DNA of the human genome. The remaining 98% of the genome exists between gene sequences (i.e., intergenic DNA sequence) and contains many important regions that are key elements to DNA replication and DNA regulatory machinery. For example, polymorphic variations in intergenic DNA sequence may influence DNA tertiary structure directly or alter binding sites of DNA regulatory machinery, including **histones** and **topoisomerases**, which exert profound influence on overall gene regulation, cellular signaling, and homeostatic responses to environmental stresses. Indeed, recent studies implicate mechanisms of DNA–histone binding in the potential underlying pathophysiology of mood disorders and drug addiction while pointing to potential therapeutic targets for novel antidepressant and antipsychotic therapies.[7] One insight that is gained when considering the size of plant and animal genomes, and the relatively small fraction of these genomes that actually encode proteins (i.e., genes), is that the retention of large noncoding regions in the genome over millions of years of generations does not appear to consume excessive cellular resources that place the organism at a disadvantage to survival and/or there is an evolutionary advantage to retaining these large noncoding regions, even those regions that do not appear to be critical for DNA replication. Note that the relevance of intergenic DNA sequence to pharmacogenetics is emerging. One potential example of these effects is that of the O^6-methylguanine DNA methyltransferase (MGMT) enzyme that repairs DNA damage induced by alkylating chemotherapeutic drugs such as temozolomide. Evidence suggests that hypermethylation of DNA regions upstream of MGMT suppress its expression in some types of B lymphoma cells, causing increased susceptibility to the cytotoxic effects of anticancer medications used in treatment.[8] However, more research and linkage studies must be carried out to fully understand how specific allelic variations in these regions will be utilized to alter drug dose and/or drug choice in clinical practice.

The human genome is made up of approximately 25,000 distinct genes, each capable of coding a unique protein, and it is these proteins that enable our cells to carry out the many different molecular, enzymatic, and mechanical processes that enable life. Because most drugs interact with proteins, pharmacogenetics deals primarily with genetic variations that affect gene regulation (i.e., DNA sequence variations that alter how much of each protein is being synthesized in the cell) and protein function or activity (i.e., DNA sequence variations in the gene that alter the amino acid sequence of the protein). Pharmacogenetics involves an understanding of how individual genetic differences in a population are the cause of variable responses to a specific dose of a drug in a population. In order to effectively examine the interactions between pharmacokinetics, pharmacodynamics, and genetics, we must first understand how genes are regulated in the cell and how the gene sequence (coding sequence) defines the primary sequence of a protein.

The simplest description of a gene's structure can be divided into (1) a regulatory region, where the cellular machinery exerts its effect on if, and how much, the gene will be "activated" or used by the cell and (2) the coding region, where the DNA sequence directly correlates with the protein sequence (see **Figure 1-1**).

The regulatory region contains specific DNA sequences and motifs where transcription factors and other regulatory elements bind, thereby promoting or preventing the transcription of the gene. During gene transcription, ribonucleic acid (RNA) polymerase binds within the regulatory region and then moves along the coding sequence to create a direct copy of the gene sequence. This RNA copy will undergo further processing before leaving the nucleus of the cell, ultimately coupling with the ribosome to synthesize the protein from the gene. In **Figure 1-2**, the details of eukaryotic transcription are described.

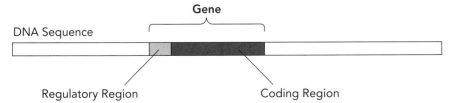

Figure 1-1 Simplified gene structure. The structure of a gene can be divided into the regulatory region, which is responsive to cellular machinery controlling its expression, and the coding region, where the DNA sequence directly correlates with the protein sequence.

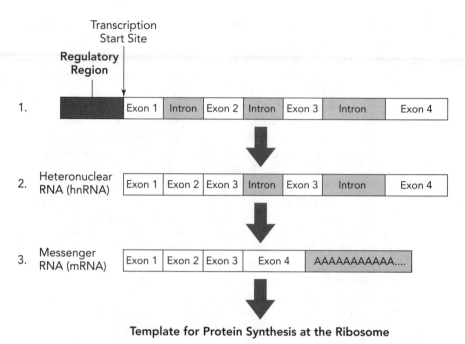

Template for Protein Synthesis at the Ribosome

Figure 1-2 Eukaryotic transcription and translation. Genetic information derived from the DNA sequence is converted to functional proteins when: beginning at the transcription start site, the double-stranded DNA sequence is directly copied into a single-stranded heteronuclear RNA (hnRNA); messenger RNA (mRNA) is formed when introns are spliced or removed from the hnRNA and a poly-A tail is added; and mRNA is translated into a protein via protein synthesis at the ribosome.

As shown in the figure, the double-stranded DNA sequence (1) is directly copied into a single-stranded RNA sequence known as heteronuclear RNA (hnRNA), beginning at the transcription start site. Heteronuclear RNA is then (2) processed by removing the **intron** regions, a process termed splicing, and (3) a poly-A tail is added, resulting in messenger RNA (mRNA), which moves from the nucleus to the ribosome for protein synthesis.

Note that the removal of the intron sequence in the hnRNA results in the concatenation of the **exon** sequences in the mRNA, which represents the coding sequence for the protein. At the ribosome, the genetic coding sequence (nucleic acids) is converted to the protein sequence (amino acids). Each and every amino acid in a protein is coded by three nucleic acids, called a **codon** (see **Figure 1-3** for a codon key). For example, the nucleic acid codon "AUG" encodes for the amino acid methionine in a protein sequence. Note that the thymine (T) in DNA is replaced by uracil (U) in RNA. In addition to the codons that encode specific amino acids, three codons (UAA, UAG,

Second Position				
	U	C	A	G	

First Position		U	C	A	G	Third Position
U	UUU – Phe UUC – Phe UUA – Leu UUG – Leu	UCU – Ser UCC – Ser UCA – Ser UCG – Ser	UAU – Tyr UAC – Tyr UAA – Stop UAG – Stop	UGU – Cys UGC – Cys UGA – Stop UGG – Trp	U C A G
C	CUU – Leu CUC – Leu CUA – Leu CUG – Leu	CCU – Pro CCC – Pro CCA – Pro CCG – Pro	CAU – His CAC – His CAA – Gln CAG – Gln	CGU – Arg CGC – Arg CGA – Arg CGG – Arg	U C A G
A	AUU – Ile AUC – Ile AUA – Ile AUG – Met	ACU – Thr ACC – Thr ACA – Thr ACG – Thr	AAU – Asn AAC – Asn AAA – Lys AAG – Lys	AGU – Ser AGC – Ser AGA – Arg AGG – Arg	U C A G
G	GUU – Val GUC – Val GUA – Val GUG – Val	GCU – Ala GCC – Ala GCA – Ala GCG – Ala	GAU – Asp GAC – Asp GAA – Glu GAG – Glu	GGU – Gly GGU – Gly GGA – Gly GGG – Gly	U C A G

Ala	Alanine	Gly	Glysine	Pro	Proline
Arg	Arginine	His	Histidine	Ser	Serine
Asn	Asparagine	Ile	Isoleucine	Thr	Threonine
Asp	Aspartic Acid	Leu	Leucine	Trp	Tryptophan
Cys	Cysteine	Lys	Lysine	Tyr	Tyrosine
Gln	Glutamine	Met	Methionine	Val	Valine
Glu	Glutamic Acid	Phe	Phenylalanine		

Figure 1-3 The genetic code. In the expression of genetic information, the codon key describes the code for each amino acid in a protein based on three nucleic acids, termed a "codon."

and UGA) encode a "stop" command, thereby stopping the growth of the protein at that point in the sequence.

Cell Biology and the Human Genome

In living systems, the cell is the basic unit of life. Each cell that contains a nucleus contains the entire genome of the organism, although the cell only utilizes a subset of genes to enable its viability and function within the organism. Within the nucleus of human cells are 23 pairs of chromosomes (46 chromosomes total). Chromosomes were originally discovered over 100 years ago using basic dyes and state-of-the-art microscopes (at that time), thus the name chromosome simply means "colored body" as a description of how they were first observed in the nucleus of the cell. One pair of chromosomes is associated with gender and is commonly referred to as the sex chromosomes. Females have two "X" sex chromosomes, whereas males have an "X" and a "Y" sex chromosome.

In simple terms, chromosomes are essentially unbroken polymers of double-stranded DNA. They often are associated with histone proteins that enable an efficient "packaging" of the DNA prior to cell division. The state of DNA in the cell correlates with the different phases of cell division (see **Figure 1-4**). It should be obvious that when a cell divides into two daughter cells, each cell must have a copy of the genome to remain viable. The cell goes through four phases to replicate itself, which includes replication of its genomic content. In the G1 phase, the activity of the cell is largely dedicated to growth and maintenance of the functions of the cell. As a cell prepares to undergo mitotic division, it enters the S phase, during which the entirety of the DNA (chromosomes) in the cell is duplicated (i.e., DNA synthesis = "S" phase), resulting in two copies of each chromosome. Completion of the DNA (chromosome) duplication leads to the G2 phase, and the

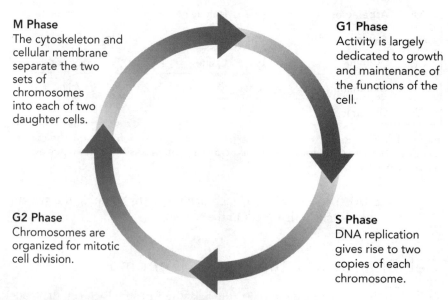

M Phase
The cytoskeleton and cellular membrane separate the two sets of chromosomes into each of two daughter cells.

G1 Phase
Activity is largely dedicated to growth and maintenance of the functions of the cell.

G2 Phase
Chromosomes are organized for mitotic cell division.

S Phase
DNA replication gives rise to two copies of each chromosome.

Figure 1-4 The four phases of the cell cycle.

chromosomes are organized in preparation for mitotic cell division. During the M phase of cell division, the cellular membrane separates the two sets of chromosomes into each of two daughter cells, and each daughter cell reenters the G1 phase, each with a complete copy of the genome within the chromosomes of its nucleus.

In addition to the chromosomal DNA found in the nucleus of the cell, a relatively small amount of DNA is found in the mitochondria. Mitochondria harbor about 16 kilobases of DNA (called mtDNA) in a circular form. In humans, the mtDNA contains 37 genes that encode proteins utilized by the mitochondria for energy production and protein synthesis. The mtDNA undergoes its own replication as mitochondria replicate within the cells of our body. Importantly, mtDNA is maternally inherited because the large female gamete (egg cell) contains hundreds of thousands of mitochondria, whereas the mtDNA in the much smaller male gamete (sperm cell) is not incorporated during fertilization of the egg. Thus, the fertilized egg only contains maternal mtDNA and is therefore used in genetic research for mapping maternal inheritance across generations.

Cells exist in the human body that do not harbor a nucleus and therefore lack a copy of the human genome. The red blood cells (RBCs, also known as erythrocytes) and platelets (also called thrombocytes) of the blood are derived from parent cells in the long bones of our bodies. Red blood cells are involved in oxygen transport in the blood and are derived from a process called erythropoiesis involving progenitor cells (e.g., proerythroblasts, polychromatic erythroblasts), whereas platelets are involved in blood clotting and are derived from megakaryocytes. These non-nucleated cells lack nuclear DNA, yet they harbor genetic information in the form of RNA, allowing the cells to synthesize proteins. The DNA that is obtained from a blood sample is actually derived from the white blood cells, which make up about 1% of blood volume in healthy adults.[9]

This is important when we consider using DNA genotyping to support advances in healthcare. If we use genotyping to screen for a neurological disease, we do not need to sample the human brain directly because almost all other cells in our body contain the complete genome. Therefore, we can carry out genotyping using cells that are easily obtainable (e.g., white blood cells, from a buccal swab to gather the cells from inside the mouth), thereby providing a noninvasive, nondestructive method for gaining access to our genomic information.

Categorically, genetic testing in humans is routinely carried out in four distinct areas: paternity and/or maternity, DNA forensics, disease predisposition, and pharmacogenetics (see **Table 1-1**). Paternity/maternity testing is used to establish a biological relationship between a parent and an offspring, whereas DNA forensics can determine the origin and/or identity of a biological sample. In both of

Table 1-1				
Categories of Human Genetic Testing				
	Paternity or Maternity Testing	**DNA Forensics**	**Disease Predisposition**	**Pharmacogenetics**
Utility	Determine biological parent.	Determine identity of crime scene DNA sample.	Determine cause of, or predisposition for, disease or disorder, or if the patient is a carrier for an inherited disease.	Predict optimal drug and/or dose for specific patient.
Sample source	Buccal swab	Varied	Buccal swab, saliva, or blood sample	Buccal swab, saliva, or blood sample
Target	Short tandem repeats (STR)	Short tandem repeats (STR)	Allelic variations linked to disease/ disorder	Genes for drug metabolism enzymes, drug transporters, and drug receptors
Rapid testing turnaround required	Infrequently	Infrequently	No	Yes

these areas, the genomic biomarkers commonly tested are called short tandem repeats, or STRs, which are short repeated sequences of DNA. Another growing area of human genomics involves testing for specific genomic biomarkers associated with disease, where the genetic cause for a disease or disorder is established as a diagnostic tool or used to determine the risk of developing the disease.

Pharmacogenetics, however, points to important distinctions among these areas of genetic testing. Each has shown tremendous utility and societal value. Yet, in order to derive the full clinical potential of genetic testing in pharmacogenetics, information regarding genetic variation as it relates to the disposition and effect of medications must be immediately available to caregivers. Thus, the value of pharmacogenetics is more likely to be dependent on technologies and information systems/procedures that allow for rapid testing and provide clinicians with more real-time access to a patient's individual genetic data.

Genetic Variation and Personalized Medicine

The essence of personalized medicine is individual genetic variation. The most obvious and perhaps most basic examples of individual genetic variation are observed outwardly. Readily apparent physical traits, such as skin tone, eye color, hair color, height, and even shoe size, are all dictated by genes that vary, in some cases dramatically, between individuals. In this sense, the gene–trait interface could be described in modern, colloquial terms as "designing" an avatar in a video game. Each player is offered choices that determine the appearance of the avatar. Analogous to a genetic menu of sorts, one can scroll through screens of options, ranging from body type to facial structure, where nuances such as the thickness of the eyebrows, shape of the nose, and distance between the eyes are presented. These choices allow an avatar to assume a uniqueness that, although immensely oversimplified, can be extrapolated to represent genetic variation and the direct relationship between genetic identity and physical traits (see **Figure 1-5**). Yet, as we move from electronic simplification to genetic reality, the avatar analogy quickly fades—the vast complexity of the human genome provides for a much deeper level of variation between individuals.

Analysis of the human genome following publication of its first complete sequence in 2003 only begins to describe this complexity. As described earlier, each human germ-line cell contains approximately three billion nucleotide base pairs of DNA comprising around 25,000 genes, and among this immense store of genetic code there is tremendous intraspecies homogeneity, a fact underscored by the discovery that all humans share roughly 99.9% of the DNA sequence.

Such uniformity makes perfect sense. Genes encode for proteins for which functions are nearly always precisely limited by their tertiary and quaternary structure, which dictates efficiency of enzymatic and/or biological processes. One dramatic example is actin, a type of cytoskeletal scaffold that owns the title of being the most abundant protein in nearly all human cells, comprising anywhere from 10–20% of total cell protein. In fact, the typical hepatocyte contains an estimated 500 million actin molecules, giving the cytosol a gel-like rather than fluid consistency.[10] As is implied by their abundance, actin proteins are essential for a variety of biological functions, such as structural integrity, cell shape, cell motility, chromosome morphology, and muscle contraction, as well as a host of intracellular events, including gene transcription and translation. Thus, it is of little surprise that the six human genes encoding for the three actin isoforms (α, β, and γ) are among the most highly conserved in the entire genome, being second only to the histone family of DNA-binding proteins. In fact, the DNA sequence of human actin is over 80% identical to that found in yeast, with a near 96% amino acid homology.[11]

This incredible degree of interspecies homogeneity means that biological activity in eukaryotes is extremely sensitive to changes in the DNA sequence. Indeed, entire clusters of genes exist with a sole recognized function of minimizing DNA mutations during

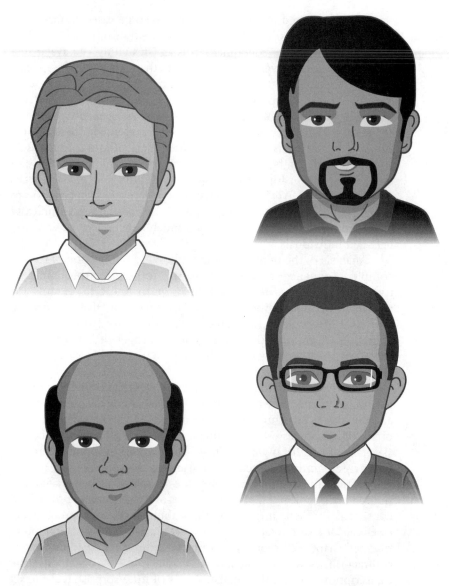

Figure 1-5 Avatars representing the authors of this text (generated by www.pickaface.net).
Source: Courtesy of Fredy Sujono from www.pickaface.net.

cell division. One such family of proteins is known as the mismatch repair genes.[12] Also highly conserved, this family of nine unique proteins "proofread" newly replicated daughter strands of DNA for relatively common errors in base incorporation by DNA polymerases, errors that would otherwise result in nearly one mutation for every 1,000 base pairs replicated. Instead, mismatch repair enzymes identify "mismatched" bases, excise them from the newly replicated daughter strand, and finally reinsert the correct deoxyribonucleotide base. This effectively reduces the average mutation rate by six orders of magnitude, or to less than one base change per billion bases.

The importance of mutation-reducing enzymatic activity is obvious. DNA sequence fidelity transmitted from parent cell to daughter and from parent organism to offspring allows for continuity of gene sequence, which provides for continuity of inherited traits. Moreover, evolutionary pressures of selection work toward maintaining individuals with as little genetic diversity as possible, at least with respect to the many thousands of genes, like those for actin, whose activity is required for sustainable life.

In spite of these Herculean cellular efforts and the constant evolutionary pressures that favor DNA fidelity across generations, genetic variation persists. Small changes in genetic code continue to arise, and these often more subtle mutations, known as polymorphisms, give rise to a deeper, and in some ways more defining, characteristic of genetic variation among individuals.

Polymorphic Genetic Variation

In the most basic sense, changes in the genetic code are observed as differences in DNA sequence called **mutations**. These changes in sequence may or may not produce observable differences in traits either in an individual or in its offspring. Mutations that occur in genomic DNA between individuals gives rise to genetic variation—that one person's DNA sequence differs from another at specific bases. Some mutations are more common than others in a population. When a particular mutation occurs in at least 1% of individuals in the population, it is commonly referred to as a **polymorphism**, which is derived literally from the Greek word meaning "many forms." For example, if at a given location in the genome 4% of individuals contain adenine (A) but the other 96% contain a cytosine (C), the A represents a polymorphism. In this way, the term polymorphism is used to help describe the prevalence of a specific genetic variation between individuals within a population.

Variants are incredibly common. Individuals differ in their DNA on average by one base pair for every 100 to 300 base pairs throughout the genome, although their frequency can be much greater within a given gene. It has been estimated that as many as 9 to 10 million polymorphisms may reside in the human genome, yet it is highly unlikely that any one individual will carry all possible polymorphic variations.[13] However, because of their frequency, polymorphisms are particularly useful in describing genetic differences between individuals, especially differences that define discrete subpopulations within the population as a whole.

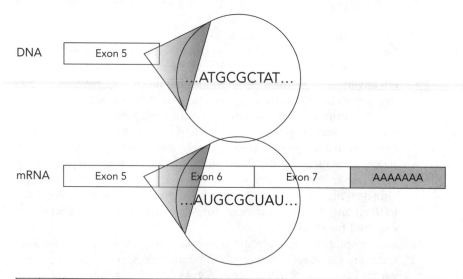

		Second Position				
		U	**C**	**A**	**G**	
First Position	**U**	UUU – Phe UUC – Phe UUA – Leu UUG – Leu	UCU – Ser UCC – Ser UCA – Ser UCG – Ser	UAU – Tyr UAC – Tyr UAA – Stop UAG – Stop	UGU – Cys UGC – Cys UGA – Stop UGG – Trp	U C A G
	C	CUU – Leu CUC – Leu CUA – Leu CUG – Leu	CCU – Pro CCC – Pro CCA – Pro CCG – Pro	CAU – His CAC – His CAA – Gin CAG – Gin	CGU – Arg CGC – Arg CGA – Arg CGG – Arg	U C A G
	A	AUU – Ile AUC – Ile AUA – Ile AUG – Met	ACU – Thr ACC – Thr ACA – Thr ACG – Thr	AAU – Asn AAC – Asn AAA – Lys AAG – Lys	AGU – Ser AGC – Ser AGA – Arg AGG – Arg	U C A G
	G	GUU – Val GUC – Val GUA – Val GUG – Val	GCU – Ala GCC – Ala GCA – Ala GCG – Ala	GAU – Asp GAC – Asp GAA – Glu GAG – Glu	GGU – Gly GGU – Gly GGA – Gly GGG – Gly	U C A G

Third Position

	Wild-Type Sequence	**Genetic Variation**
mRNA	…ACC—GCC—UAU…	…ACC—UCC—UAU…
Protein Activity	…Thr—Ala—Tyr…	…Thr—Ser—Tyr…
Clinical Outcome	Normal binding to β-myosin	Reduced β-myosin binding
	Normal cardiac muscle contraction	Decreased cardiac muscle contraction and clinical symptoms of left ventricular hypertrophy

The manifestation of variation in the genetic code can be dramatic. One such example is found in the human α-actin gene. Familial hypertrophic cardiomyopathy (FHC) is an autosomal dominant congenital disease that leads to compromised cardiac function (syncope, angina, arrhythmias, and heart failure) and is the leading cause of sudden death in young people.[14] At least nine different mutations in α-actin have been directly linked to FHC, including a guanine to thymine (G→T) mutation at base 253 of exon 5 in the actin gene. This change, where the **wild-type** or typical sequence found in "normal" individuals is altered, results in the substitution of the amino acid serine for alanine at position 295 within the actin protein and is denoted as Ala295Ser. The simple G→T variation results in an actin molecule whose binding affinity for β-myosin is diminished, which reduces the strength of cardiac muscle contraction and can contribute to potentially fatal hypertrophy of the left ventricle (see **Figure 1-6**).[15]

Understandably, potentially serious physiological consequences that can be expressed at a young age make the actin Ala295Ser variation less likely to be transmitted generationally. However, a far greater degree of genetic variation is interspersed throughout the genome. Remember that nearly 99% of the genome is contained within regions of DNA considered noncoding or intergenic that do not directly encode for protein. Thus, the vast majority of variations are likely to be neither harmful nor beneficial per se. Yet, there is a growing appreciation for the potential role of polymorphisms in directly causing, or indirectly associating with, characteristics and traits that vary between groups within a population, especially as it pertains to individual responses to drugs.

In general, polymorphisms can be categorized into two main types: **single nucleotide polymorphisms**, commonly referred to as **SNPs** (pronounced "snips"), and insertions or deletions, commonly referred to as **indels**, with each category further differentiated into subcategories based on the nature, location, and effect of the polymorphism.

The most common type of polymorphism in pharmacogenetics is the SNP (see **Figure 1-7**). Single nucleotide polymorphisms are polymorphisms that occur at a single nucleotide where any one of the four bases of DNA (A, C, G, and T) may be substituted for another. An estimated 90% of all genetic variation in the human genome is thought to

Figure 1-6 Variation in the human cardiac α-actin gene associated with familial hypertrophic cardiomyopathy (FHC). A guanine to thymine (G→T) mutation in exon 5 of the human cardiac α-actin gene results in variation in the mRNA codon sequence and subsequent mistranslation of serine at amino acid position 295 rather than alanine. The resulting actin molecule exhibits reduced binding affinity for β-myosin, resulting in diminished cardiac muscle contraction and clinical symptoms associated with hypertrophy of the left ventricle.

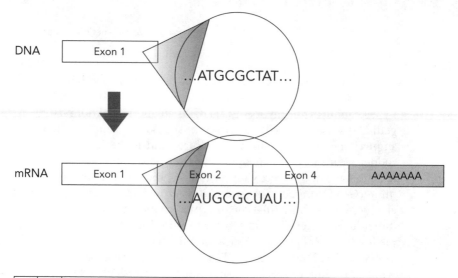

		Second Position				
		U	C	A	G	
First Position	U	UUU – Phe UUC – Phe UUA – Leu UUG – Leu	UCU – Ser UCC – Ser UCA – Ser UCG – Ser	UAU – Tyr UAC – Tyr UAA – Stop UAG – Stop	UGU – Cys UGC – Cys UGA – Stop UGG – Trp	U C A G
	C	CUU – Leu CUC – Leu CUA – Leu CUG – Leu	CCU – Pro CCC – Pro CCA – Pro CCG – Pro	CAU – His CAC – His CAA – Gln CAG – Gln	CGU – Arg CGC – Arg CGA – Arg CGG – Arg	U C A G
	A	AUU – Ile AUC – Ile AUA – Ile AUG – Met	ACU – Thr ACC – Thr ACA – Thr ACG – Thr	AAU – Asn AAC – Asn AAA – Lys AAG – Lys	AGU – Ser AGC – Ser AGA – Arg AGG – Arg	U C A G
	G	GUU – Val GUC – Val GUA – Val GUG – Val	GCU – Ala GCC – Ala GCA – Ala GCG – Ala	GAU – Asp GAC – Asp GAA – Glu GAG – Glu	GGU – Gly GGU – Gly GGA – Gly GGG – Gly	U C A G

(Third Position)

	Wild-Type Sequence	Synonymous SNP	Nonsynonymous SNP
mRNA Codon Sequence	...AUG—CGC—UAU...	...AUG—CGA—UAU...	...AUG—AGC—UAU...
Protein Sequence	...Met—Arg—Tyr...	...Met—Arg—Tyr...	...Met—Ser—Tyr...

Figure 1-7 Synonymous and nonsynonymous SNPs. Synonymous, or sense, SNPs are changes to a single nucleotide that alter the mRNA codon sequence without changes to the translated protein. In this hypothetical example, a cytosine to adenine (C → A) polymorphism changes the codon from CGC to CGA, but both codons are translated to arginine. In contrast, nonsynonymous, or missense, SNPs are changes to a single nucleotide that result in altered mRNA codon sequence and subsequent mistranslation of the protein. In this case, a cytosine to adenine (C → A) polymorphism results in the translation of a serine rather than arginine.

be derived from SNPs. Interestingly, the substitution of C $\rightarrow$ T constitutes roughly two out of every three SNPs.[13] Single nucleotide polymorphisms can be located in either coding or noncoding regions of DNA. Recall that coding regions contained within the genes make up less than 2% of the total DNA in the genome. As a result of the relative paucity of bases that make up this region, SNPs in coding regions occur less frequently than SNPs in noncoding regions but have a far greater potential to influence the phenotype of an individual. In this sense, the old colloquialism "location, location, location" certainly applies to SNPs.

Single nucleotide polymorphisms with the most direct genetic influence are located within the coding region of DNA. These polymorphisms are classified as either synonymous (also called sense mutations), which result in translation of the same amino acid, or nonsynonymous (also called missense mutations), which result in translation of a different amino acid. Another type of coding SNP can be classified as a nonsense mutation in that the polymorphism results in the inappropriate insertion of a stop codon in the growing mRNA, ultimately leading to a truncated protein product. In these ways, SNPs may cause important differences in gene function and/or expression. For example, mRNA transcripts used for translation can be directly altered by SNPs, leading to compromised transcript stability or altered RNA splicing. Likewise, coding nonsynonymous or nonsense SNPs may influence protein structure, stability, substrate affinities, and so on.

Apolipoprotein E (ApoE), a gene associated with Alzheimer's disease, can serve as an example of the effects of nonsynonymous SNPs located in the coding region of a gene.[16] Apolipoprotein E is a member of a family of proteins whose function is to bind to and assist in the transport of lipids in the circulatory system and is the predominant lipoprotein in the brain. Two SNPs, both thymine to cytosine (T$\rightarrow$C) substitutions, are located within ApoE that result in the translation of more basic arginine residues at amino acid positions 112 and 158 instead of neutral cysteines. These changes, when found together, are known as the ApoE ε4 allele and transform ApoE into an isoform that exhibits increased binding affinity to amyloid β, a small protein involved in the pathology of Alzheimer's disease.[17] Apolipoprotein ε4 is found in high abundance in neurofibrillary tangles characteristic of Alzheimer's disease.[17] In fact, the SNPs associated with the ApoE ε4 allele, which occur in 5% of the population, are now considered to be the single greatest genetic risk factor for the development of Alzheimer's disease, which is the leading cause of senile dementia in the elderly and effects nearly 25 million adults worldwide.

Importantly, the influence of SNPs is not limited to those found directly in coding regions. At least one important function of noncoding DNA is to regulate the expression of mRNA transcripts. Thus, noncoding polymorphisms located in regulatory regions, including promoters, areas of DNA that respond to cellular machinery that

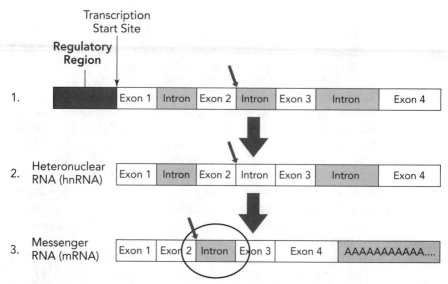

Figure 1-8 The potential impact of noncoding SNPs. SNPs located in noncoding regions of DNA, such as promoters, introns, and the boundary between exons and introns, can result in altered splicing and/or expression of mRNA transcripts. In this example, the SNP located at the proximal intronic boundary between exons 2 and 3 (indicated by arrows) alters the DNA sequence recognized by splicing machinery within the cell, eliminating the splice site. The resulting mRNA transcript erroneously retains the intron, leading to translation of the intron sequence into an altered protein product.

control gene expression, introns, and the boundary between exons and introns, lead to potential changes in transcription factor binding, mRNA transcript stability, or RNA splicing (see **Figure 1-8**).[18]

It is worth noting, not without irony, that there is considerable variation in the nomenclature used to describe genetic variation. Frequently, the same polymorphisms are described by different names in various basic science and clinical sources in the literature. For instance, a hypothetical single-base variation from adenine to thymine could be designated as A→T, A/T, A>T, or even A123T or 123A>T to denote base position within the gene. Making matters even more confusing, early studies of polymorphisms did not benefit from the standardized DNA sequence databases that exist today, such as the National Center for Biotechnology Information, or NCBI (www.ncbi.nlm.nih .gov). Rather, investigators studying identical regions of DNA frequently used sequences or fragments of DNA with different starting points relative to the actual genomic sequence. Thus, studies of our hypothetical polymorphism at position 123 could appear in the literature as A123T in one study and A323T in another if the sequence used in the latter began 200 bases upstream relative to that used in the former.

Although it will likely take some time for standardized nomenclature to take hold in the literature, recent efforts have produced several proposals for a systematic methodology of SNP nomenclature.

One prominent example is from the Human Genome Variation Society.[19] Its recommendations for the naming of human sequence variation promote a basic system focusing on first naming the gene of interest followed by designating the level of sequence variation: at the level of DNA, located in either coding regions designated as "c," genomic or noncoding regions as "g," or mitochondrial regions as "m." This nomenclature is not to be confused with the molecular biological term complementary DNA, which also is designated cDNA, and is likewise derived from reverse transcribing messenger RNA, or mRNA, so that only exons are included in the sequence. Thus, a coding reference sequence represents only DNA information contained in processed mRNA, whereas gDNA sequences represent DNA information identical to how it exists in the genome, containing DNA from introns, exons, and intergenic regions. Ribonucleic acid and protein sequence variation are respectively designated by "r." or "p." Actual variation in a sequence is described by listing first the reference or wild-type sequence/base followed by the sequence variation. Thus, applying this nomenclature system, the α-actin variation already described would be named c.253G>T to indicate the variation of sequence at position 253 in the coding reference sequence in the α-actin gene where the reference base guanine has been replaced by the variant thymine. This naming system could further be applied to describe the resulting change in terms of base substitution at the protein level using p.295S>A or p.295Ser>Ala where the serine at amino acid position 295 in the α-actin protein is changed to alanine.

Another SNP nomenclature system that is widely used is the **reference sequence number**, or the **refSNP**, **rs#**, or **rs**. Developed for use in the Single Nucleotide Polymorphism Database (dbSNP) hosted by the NCBI, this system is designed to reference genetic variation such as SNPs according to more precise locations within the genome rather than the arbitrary and varying segments of DNA frequently used in individual studies.[20] This is akin to providing each SNP with an exact chromosomal street address, where possible, that is used to define the SNP. For instance, rs113513162 is the specific, consistent identifier in dbSNP for the c.253G>T actin mutation in exon 5 of the ACTC gene located on chromosome 15. Efforts such as these that normalize the nomenclature and referencing of variation in the genetic code have proven valuable in decreasing the incidence of ambiguous or misleading literature references to SNPs.

Genetic variation can also be described at the whole-gene level. Perhaps the most relevant example for the purposes of this text is that of the human cytochrome (CYP) P450 genes for which gene-wide variation is defined by well-accepted nomenclature.[21] In this system, the superfamily designation of "CYP" precedes that given for family (indicated by number), subfamily (indicated by letter), and individual subfamily member (again indicated by number). Importantly, allelic differences are defined by a number or a number and a letter following an asterisk (*) designation. It is important to note that in this nomenclature system the "*1" designation most commonly refers to the wild-type gene, whereas integers of "2" or greater denote polymorphic alleles typically numbered in order of their discovery and validation. For some genes, the nomenclature also includes the designation of "*1A" as the wild-type and "*1B," "*1C," "*1D," and so on as variants.

All told, this system allows for genotypic variation, in some cases involving multiple SNPs, to be described in phenotypic terms by referencing differences in an allele rather than a nucleotide. For example, CYP2C9 is a primary metabolizing enzyme of drugs, including the antiseizure medication phenytoin, the anticoagulant warfarin, and many nonsteroidal anti-inflammatory drugs, such as naproxen. A SNP that occurs within the CYP2C9 gene resulting in a cytosine to thymine (C→T; rs1799853) conversion leads to decreased enzymatic function. This allelic polymorphism is designated by CYP2C9*2 and is used to denote individuals susceptible to elevated drug levels following administration of typical doses of these medications (see **Figure 1-9**).

The other major category of polymorphism is indels. This genetic variation involves the insertion or deletion of DNA either as single nucleotides or as two or more nucleotides, in some cases spanning regions of DNA encompassing an entire gene. One of the best characterized forms of indels is the duplication of the cytochrome P450 drug metabolizing enzyme CYP2D6, where individuals have been

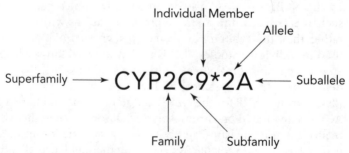

Figure 1-9 Nomenclature for the cytochrome P-450 (CYP) alleles. The established nomenclature system for alleles of the cytochrome P-450 (CYP) superfamily designates "CYP" followed by family number, subfamily letter, and individual subfamily number. Allelic differences are defined by number or a number and letter following an asterisk (*).

found to possess as many as 13 copies of the gene. In contrast, GSTT1, a gene encoding for the glutathione-conjugating enzyme glutathione S-transferase theta-1, is entirely deleted in some individuals, which sometimes leads to reduced metabolism of **xenobiotics**, particularly those with electrophillic and hydrophobic properties.[22] In this case, the existence of alternative metabolic pathways for some compounds means that the phenotypic effect of this gene deletion may not be observed.

A classic example of the pharmacogenetic consequences of polymorphic variation can be found in a family member of the cytochrome P450 enzymes, CYP2D6. Located on chromosome 22, CYP2D6 is a primary mechanism for the metabolism of nearly 100 drugs, including many antidepressants, such as fluoxetine; many neuroleptics, such as haloperidol; beta blockers, such as propanolol; and analgesics, such as codeine. Individuals carrying the wild-type alleles for CYP2D6 (CYP2D6*1) are phenotypically considered extensive metabolizers (EM) in that substrates at CYP2D6, such as the drugs aforementioned, are metabolized efficiently.[23] If one were to compare CYP2D6 metabolic activity to the volume dial on a stereo, the CYP2D6*1 allele would be analogous to a normal setting (see **Figure 1-10**).

Most of the clinically relevant CYP2D6 SNPs identified thus far result in diminished enzymatic activity associated with poor metabolizer (PM) or intermediate metabolizer (IM) phenotypes. For example, the CYP2D6*4 allele containing the 1846G>A polymorphism is a splicing defect in CYP2D6 that results in a truncated, nonfunctional protein product.[24] It is among the most common CYP2D6 SNPs found in Caucasian populations accounting for a significant percentage of mutant alleles. Another example of the PM phenotype is the CYP2D6*10 allele containing the 100C>T SNP, which results in diminished enzymatic activity via enhanced protein degradation.[25] It is the most common CYP-related polymorphism found in Asian populations (nearly 50% of individuals), whereas the CYP2D6*4 allele is seen at a much lower frequency in this group. Among individuals of African ethnicity, the CYP2D6*17 allele containing the 1023C>T polymorphism is most common, resulting in a deficiency of hydrolase activity due to reduced substrate-binding affinity.[26]

Evidence also suggests indel polymorphic expression of CYP2D6. Repetition of a 42-kilobase DNA fragment containing CYP2D6*2 results in CYP2D6 duplication that is phenotypically expressed as an ultrarapid metabolizer (UM) phenotype.[27] In fact, as many as 13 copies of the enzyme have been indentified in one individual's genome. Interestingly, this phenomenon is thought to have arisen from selective pressures associated with specific geographic regions. The incidence of CYP2D6 duplication has been reported with a frequency of less than 2% in Asians and less than 5% in Western Europeans but as much as 16% in Ethiopians.[28,29] Thus, the frequency of individuals possessing CYP2D6

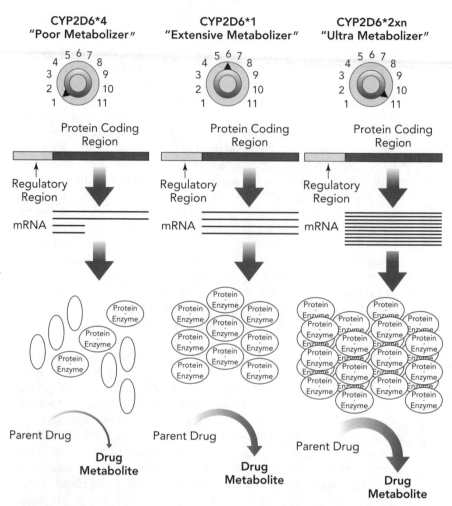

Figure 1-10 Genotypic and phenotypic differences in CYP2D6 metabolism. Individuals carrying the wild-type alleles for CYP2D6 (CYP2D6*1) are phenotypically considered "extensive metabolizers." Carriers of the CYP2D6*4 allele containing the 1846G>A polymorphism produce a truncated, nonfunctional protein product and therefore exhibit a "poor metabolizer" phenotype. The CYP2D6*2xn allele indicates repetition of a 42-kilobase DNA fragment, resulting in CYP2D6 duplication that is phenotypically expressed as an "ultrarapid metabolizer" phenotype.

duplication suggests a geographical gradient, possibly resulting from dietary pressures where, historically speaking, the detoxification capacity afforded by CYP2D6 duplication may have been essential for African diets relative to more European-based diets.

Fascinating though they may be from purely anthropological and genetic viewpoints, these observations have profound clinical implications. First, for each of these groups, individuals possessing PM CYP2D6 polymorphisms may require reduced dosing of substrate drugs in order to avoid toxicities associated with decreased drug metabolism, which in many cases can be severe or even fatal. In contrast, individuals possessing CYP2D6 UM polymorphisms may require the polar opposite therapeutic course, that of increased rather than decreased dosing, in order to avoid symptoms associated with drug inefficacy. Second, these examples highlight the potential for pharmacogenetics to provide a mechanistic basis as to why individuals belonging to specific ethnic groups may respond very differently to standard drug therapy and eventually may provide a means for personalized dosing of those medications in advance. At the same time, these findings should provide ample caution against making assumptions based on ethnic background when treating individual patients. Remember, personalized medicine deals with using individual genetic information to support clinical decision making for optimal patient care. Ideally, increased prevalence of a pharmacogenetically relevant SNP in an ethnic population affords valuable consideration, but not a conclusion, at least not without genetic data specific to the individual patient.

Consider the therapeutic challenge of treating a patient with a needed medication whose primary metabolism occurs via CYP2D6, all while facing the unknown possibility that the patient's metabolic capacity could range anywhere from PM status to UM status. With this perspective, it is hardly surprising that according to the U.S. Food and Drug Administration nearly one million adverse drug reactions are reported each year in the United States, half of which lead to serious patient outcomes such as hospitalization or disability and almost 100,000 directly result in death.[30] Clearly, not all of these adverse events are attributable to pharmacogenetic influences. Many are undoubtedly the result of human error, such as administering the incorrect dose contrary to a correctly prescribed regimen. However, it ought to give one pause to realize that many adverse events are attributable not to human error, but to errors in humans. Or, in other words, adverse events arise not just when incorrect medications and/or doses are administered, but also when they are correctly prescribed and administered to individuals whose pharmacogenetic profiles may contraindicate such therapy.

In spite of these examples of dramatic phenotypes of polymorphic variation between individuals, it is more common that a pharmacogenetic trait cannot be clearly associated with a single SNP or indel. In this case, haplotypes can sometimes be used to associate **genotype** with phenotype. In true genetic terms, a **haplotype** refers to regions of DNA, such as a combination of alleles, that are inherited but that may or may not determine phenotype traits. Haplotypes are relatively common. It has been estimated that most genes contain between 2 and 53 haplotypes, with an average of 14. A haplotype has been frequently used to describe groups of SNPs that are inherited together. Haplotypes themselves may not have a direct effect on drug response, but their proximity to an unidentified causative mutation may allow them to act as a marker for a particular drug response.

One example of the use of haplotypes in predicting individual drug responses is found in the β_2 adrenergic receptor (β_2AR).[31] Twelve haplotypes have been identified in the 5′ untranslated region (UTR) and in the coding region of the *ADRB2* gene that encodes for the β_2AR receptor. Several of these haplotypes have been associated with a greater than two fold increase in response to the β_2AR agonist albuterol, which is the prototypical agent in the class of sympathomimetic drugs used as first-line bronchodilators in treating symptoms of both asthma and chronic obstructive pulmonary disease (COPD). Importantly, no individual SNPs located within the haplotypes were able to be causatively linked to improved β_2AR-mediated bronchodilation. Thus, both SNPs and haplotypes can be used to map genetic changes that are associated with an individualized drug response.

The examples provided thus far show a direct link between genotype and phenotype—between the specific genetic makeup of an individual and the response of the individual to a drug. However, establishing an association between a genetic polymorphism and a specific drug response is more complicated when multiple polymorphisms within a gene and/or multiple genes are involved.

This is most easily discussed when considering traits that are **monogenic**, or those derived from a single gene. For example, each individual inherits two alleles of CYP2C9 (one from mom and one from dad). Therefore, the overall activity of CYP2C9 results from the combined contribution of both alleles. By definition, most individuals inherit two wild-type copies of CYP2C9, which means that most of us exhibit "normal" metabolic activity of the enzyme. However, what if an individual inherits the wild-type CYP2C9 allele from one parent but the CYP2C9*2 polymorphism from the other parent? In this case, the individual would be considered **heterozygous** for CYP2C9 (written CYP2C9*1/*2) in that he or she possesses two different alleles for the same gene, one fully functional and the other with compromised enzymatic activity. If both alleles were to contain the CYP2C9*2 polymorphism, the individual would be considered **homozygous** (CYP2C9*2/*2), resulting in greatly diminished metabolism by the CYP2C9 enzyme. Thus, one would expect to see a graded loss of metabolism across individuals who are wild-type (CYP2C9*1/*1), heterozygous (CYP2C9*1/*2), and homozygous (CYP2C9*2/*2) for the CYP2C9*2 polymorphism. This is referred to as a gene-dose response relationship (see **Figure 1-11**).

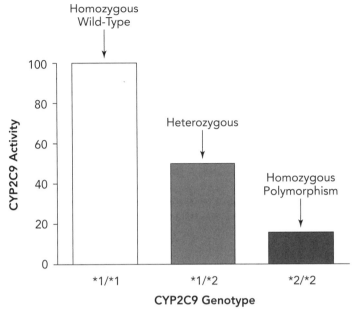

Figure 1-11 Allelic expression of CYP2C9*2 polymorphisms as an example of a monogenic trait. CYP2C9 activity results from the combined contribution of both alleles. Most individuals carry two alleles of the wild-type CYP2C9*1 and therefore exhibit full metabolic activity of the enzyme. Individuals who inherit one wild-type CYP2C9*1 allele and one polymorphic CYP2C9*2 allele are considered heterozygous for CYP2C9 and exhibit diminished enzymatic activity. If both alleles are the CYP2C9*2 polymorphism, the individual would be considered homozygous for the polymorphism, resulting in greatly diminished metabolism via CYP2C9.

In this simplistic example, the phenotype of CYP2C9 activity can be explained by the direct relationship between trait and genotype. But what if we expand our analysis to consider not just CYP2C9 activity but the overall response to a drug metabolized by the enzyme?

As an anticoagulant, warfarin has been used extensively to prevent thromboembolism but is limited in use by a narrow therapeutic index. Inadequate drug therapy increases the likelihood of potentially fatal thrombolytic events, whereas toxicity may result in life-threatening hemorrhaging. The anticoagulant effects of warfarin are mediated by inhibition of vitamin K epoxide reductase complex subunit 1 (VKORC1), a key factor in the clotting process.[32,33] Thus, the warfarin response is dependent on the function of its drug target, VKORC1, and its metabolizing enzyme, CYP2C9. Importantly, polymorphisms have been identified in VKORC1, including a guanine to adenine conversion (−1639G>A; rs9923231) that increases an individual's sensitivity to warfarin.[34,35] This means there exist subpopulations of patients that carry the CYP2C9*2 polymorphism, the −1639G>A VKORC1 polymorphism, or both. Moreover, each individual will be either heterozygous or homozygous for each polymorphism, with each polymorphism potentially altering the anticoagulant response to warfarin.

This more intricate scenario describes a **multigenic trait** where the phenotypic expression of the trait (in this case the anticoagulant response to warfarin) is dependent upon the function of several genes rather than just one. As complicated as this may appear, this gene–gene interaction still greatly oversimplifies the actual clinical condition. Consider that the warfarin response is influenced by not just two genes (gene–drug interactions) but rather the confluence of many more factors, such as age, weight, and sex, which are further compounded by other environmental variables (gene–environment interactions), such as concurrent drug therapy, and behavioral choices, such as smoking or diet. Merely attempting to approximate such complexity helps to highlight the complicated relationship that can exist between a drug response and genotype.

Review Questions

1. Pharmacogenomics is the study of the relationship between genetic variation and drug response.
   a. True
   b. False

2. Genetic variation in the nucleotide sequence of DNA necessarily results in changes in amino acid sequence and protein functionality.
   a. True
   b. False

3. In describing genetic variation, mutations and polymorphisms can be differentiated by which of the following?
   a. Frequency of the variation
   b. Functional effects of the variation
   c. Location of the variation within the genome
   d. Mutations and polymorphisms are indistinguishable

4. A coding synonymous single nucleotide polymorphism is most likely to induce a change in which of the following?
   a. Enzyme–substrate affinity
   b. Receptor–ligand binding
   c. RNA splicing
   d. Transcription

5. Which of the following metabolic enzymes is associated with both poor metabolizer (PM) and ultrarapid metabolizer (UM) phenotypes?
   a. NADP
   b. CYP2D6
   c. TPMT
   d. VKORC1

6. Which of the following CYP2D6 polymorphisms is an example of an indel?
   a. CYP2D6*4
   b. CYP2D6*2
   c. CYP2D6*10
   d. CYP2D6*17

7. Which of the following is the best description of a haplotype?
   a. A common mutation in DNA in a given population observed at greater than 1% frequency.
   b. An observable characteristic or trait.
   c. A series of polymorphisms that are inherited together.
   d. Possessing two different alleles for the same trait.

8. Polymorphisms such as those found in CYP2C9 result in heterozygous individuals who often display intermediate enzyme activity and wild-type and homozygous individuals who display either fully functional or nonfunctional enzyme activity, respectively. This trimodal phenotype is indicative of which of the following?
   a. A monogenic trait
   b. A multigenic trait
   c. Neither A nor B
   d. It is not possible to tell.

9. A patient who recently started taking the antipsychotic medication haloperidol presents with dry mouth, restlessness, spasms of the neck muscles, and weight gain, all of which are adverse effects associated with haloperidol toxicity. Based on your knowledge of the pharmacogenetic influence of CYP polymorphisms, you speculate that this patient is:
   a. homozygous for the CYP2D6*4 allele.
   b. homozygous for the CYP2D6*2xn allele.
   c. homozygous for the VKCOR1 (AA) allele.
   d. homozygous for the CYP2C9*1 allele.

References

1. PharmGKB. Questions about pharmacogenomics: What is the difference between pharmacogenetics and pharmacogenomics? Available at: www.pharmgkb.org/resources/faqs.jsp. Accessed August 21, 2012.

2. International Human Genome Sequencing Consortium. Initial sequencing and analysis of the human genome. *Nature.* 2001;409(6822):860–921.

3. Greilhuber J, Volleth M, Loidl J. Genome size of man and animals relative to the plant *Allium cepa. Can J Genet Cytol.* 1983;25(6):554–560.

4. Lim K-B, Chung J-D, van Kronenburg B, et al. Introgression of Lilium *rubellum* Baker chromosomes into L. *longiflorum* Thunb: Agenome painting study of the F1 hybrid, BC1 and BC2 progenies. *Chromosome Res.* 2000;8:119–125.

5. Hallen HE, Luo H, Scott-Craig JS, Walton JD. Gene family encoding the major toxins of lethal *Amanita* mushrooms. *Proc Natl Acad Sci.* 2007;104(48):19097–19101.

6. Sauvain-Dugerdil C, Léridon H, Mascie-Taylor CGN. Human *clocks: The bio-cultural meanings of age.* New York: Peter Lang; 2006.

7. Covington HE, Maze I, LaPlant QC, et al. Antidepressant actions of histone deacetylase inhibitors. *J Neurosci.* 2009;29(37):11451–11460.

8. Rabik CA, Njoku MC, Dolan ME. Inactivation of O^6-alkylguanine DNA alkyltransferase as a means to enhance chemotherapy. *Cancer Treat Rev.* 2006;32(4):261–276.

9. Alberts B, Johnson A, Lewis J. Leukocyte functions and percentage breakdown. In: Alberts B (ed.). *Molecular biology of the cell.* 4th ed. New York: Garland Science; 2002.

10. Lodish H, Berk A, Matsudaira P, et al. Microfilaments and intermediate filaments. In: Lodish H, Berk A, Zipursky SL, Matsudaira P, Baltimore D, Darnell J (eds.). *Molecular cell biology.* New York: W.H. Freeman; 2004.

11. Vandekerckhove J, Weber K. At least six different actins are expressed in a higher mammal: An analysis based on the amino acid sequence of the amino-terminal tryptic peptide. *J Mol Biol.* 1978;126:783–802.

12. Iyer RR, Pluciennik A, Burdett V, Modrich PL. DNA mismatch repair: Functions and mechanisms. *Chem Rev.* 2006;106:302–323.

13. Chakravarti A. To a future of genetic medicine. *Nature.* 2001;409:822–823.

14. Maron BJ. Hypertrophic cardiomyopathy: A systematic review. *JAMA.* 2002;287:1308–1320.

15. Mogensen J, Klausen IC, Pedersen AK, et al. Alpha-cardiac actin is a novel disease gene in familial hypertrophic cardiomyopathy. *J Clin Invest.* 1999;103:R39–R43.

16. Cacabelos R, Martinez R, Fernandez-Novoa L, et al. Genomics of dementia. *Int J Alzheimers Dis.* 2012;2012:1–37.

17. Corder EH, Saunders AM, Strittmatter WJ, et al. Gene dose of apolipoprotein E type 4 allele and the risk of Alzheimer's disease in late onset families. *Science.* 1993;261:921–923.

18. Zhang W, Huang RS, Dolan ME. Integrating epigenomics into pharmacogenomic studies. *Pharmgenomics Pers Med.* 2008;2008(1):7–14.

19. den Dunnen JT, Antonarakis SE. Human Genome Variation Society. Recommendations for the description of sequence variants. *Hum Mutat.* 2000;15:7–12.

20. National Center for Biotechnology Information. dbSNP Short Genetic Variations. Available at: www.ncbi.nlm.nih.gov/projects/SNP. Accessed August 21, 2012.

21. Ingelman-Sundberg M, Daly AK, Oscarson M, Nebert DW. Human cytochrome P450 (CYP) genes: Recommendations for the nomenclature of alleles. *Pharmacogenetics.* 2000;10:91–93.

22. Sprenger R, Schlagenhaufer R, Kerb R, et al. Characterization of the glutathione S-transferase GSTT1 deletion: Discrimination of all genotypes by polymerase chain reaction indicates a trimodular genotype-phenotype correlation. *Pharmacogenetics.* 2000;10:557–565.

23. Kimura S, Umeno M, Skoda RC, et al. The human debrisoquine 4-hydroxylase (CYP2D) locus: Sequence and identification of the polymorphic CYP2D6 gene, a related gene, and a pseudogene. *Am J Hum Genet.* 1989;45:889–904.

24. Kagimoto M, Heim M, Kagimoto K, et al. Multiple mutations of the human cytochrome P450IID6 gene (CYP2D6) in poor metabolizers of debrisoquine: Study of the functional significance of individual mutations by expression of chimeric genes. *J Biol Chem.* 1990;265:17209–17214.

25. Yokota H, Tamura S, Furuya H, et al. Evidence for a new variant CYP2D6 allele CYP2D6J in a Japanese population associated with lower in vivo rates of sparteine metabolism. *Pharmacogenetics.* 1993;3:256–263.

26. Masimirembwa C, Persson I, Bertilsson L, et al. A novel mutant variant of the CYP2D6 gene (CYP2D6*17) common in a black African population: Association with diminished debrisoquine hydroxylase activity. *Br J Clin Pharmacol.* 1996;42:713–719.

27. Johansson I, Lundqvist E, Bertilsson L, et al. Inherited amplification of an active gene in the cytochrome P450 CYP2D locus as a cause of ultrarapid metabolism of debrisoquine. *Proc Natl Acad Sci.* 1993;90:11825–11829.

28. Bradford LD. CYP2D6 allele frequency in European Caucasians, Asians, Africans and their descendants. *Pharmacogenomics.* 2002;3:229–243.

29. Ingelman-Sundberg M. Genetic polymorphisms of cytochrome P450 2D6 (CYP2D6): Clinical consequences, evolutionary aspects, and functional diversity. *Pharmacogenomics J.* 2005;5:6–13.

30. U.S. Food and Drug Administration. Adverse Event Reporting System (AERS). Available at: www.fda.gov/Drugs/GuidanceComplianceRegulatoryInformation /Surveillance/AdverseDrugEffects/default.htm. Accessed August 20, 2012.

31. Drysdale CM, McGraw DW, Stack CB, et al. Complex promoter and coding region beta 2-adrenergic receptor haplotypes alter receptor expression and predict in vivo responsiveness. *Proc Natl Acad Sci.* 2000;97:10483–10488.

32. Higashi MK, Veenstra DL, Kondo LM, et al. Association between CYP2C9 genetic variants and anticoagulation-related outcomes during warfarin therapy. *JAMA.* 2002;287:1690–1698.

33. Li T, Chang CY, Jin DY, et al. Identification of the gene for vitamin K epoxide reductase. *Nature.* 2004;427:541–544.

34. Veenstra DL, Blough DK, Higashi MK, et al. CYP2C9 haplotype structure in European American warfarin patients and association with clinical outcomes. *Clin Pharmacol Ther.* 2005;77:353–364.

35. Wadelius M, Chen LY, Downes K, et al. Common VKORC1 and GGCX polymorphisms associated with warfarin dose. *Pharmacogenomics J.* 2005; 5:262–270.

Pharmacogenetics Related to Pharmacokinetics and Pharmacodynamics

Section II presents the interface between pharmacogenetics and pharmacokinetics and pharmacogenetics and pharmacodynamics as underlying concepts influencing a drug's concentration-time profile and concentration-effect relationship(s). This section relates genetic influences on pharmacokinetics and pharmacodynamics in a conceptual and mathematical sense.

Chapter 2

Pharmacogenetics and Pharmacokinetics

LEARNING OBJECTIVES

Upon completion of this chapter, the student will be able to:

1. Recognize the influence of genetic polymorphisms on the absorption, distribution, metabolism, and excretion of drugs.
2. Differentiate, based on genetic polymorphisms, cytochrome P450 poor metabolizers, intermediate metabolizers, extensive metabolizers, and ultrarapid metabolizers relative to the absorption, distribution, metabolism, and excretion of drugs.
3. Explain how a specific genetic polymorphism would affect the design of a patient's drug dosing regimen.
4. Differentiate between influx and efflux transporters relative to tissue location and influence on the absorption, distribution, metabolism, and excretion of drugs.
5. Propose alterations to a patient's dosing regimen based on the pharmacogenetic influence on absorption, distribution, metabolism, and excretion.

41

The student should demonstrate an understanding of how drug metabolizing enzymes and drug transporters are influenced by genetic variation. The student should also understand that variation in these proteins results in variation in pharmacokinetics, which can influence how a person absorbs, distributes, metabolizes, and excretes a given drug, all in the context of the patient's response to the drug.

Key Terms	
absorption rate constant (k_a; time^{-1})	The rate constant representing the first-order absorption of a drug from an extravascular site (e.g., the gastrointestinal tract).
area under the curve (AUC; amt/vol · time)	A measure of drug exposure as the integrated area under the plasma drug concentration versus time curve from time zero to infinity.
bioavailability (F)	The rate and extent of drug absorption; the fraction of the dose reaching systemic circulation unchanged.
clearance (CL; vol/time)	The volume of biologic fluid from which drug is removed per unit time.
cytochrome P450 (CYP)	A superfamily of oxidative metabolic enzymes.
efflux transporter	A protein that moves drug out of cells/tissues.
elimination rate constant (k_e; time^{-1})	The rate constant representing the first-order elimination of drug.
extensive metabolizer (EM)	An individual with two "normal-function" alleles relative to a drug metabolizing enzyme.
genotype	The specific set of alleles inherited at a locus on a given gene.
intermediate metabolizer (IM)	In general, an individual with one "loss-of-function" allele and one "normal–function" allele relative to a drug metabolizing enzyme.
loading dose (D_L; amt)	The initial dose of a drug administered with the intent of producing a near steady-state average concentration.
maximum concentration (C_{max}; amt/vol)	The highest concentration of drug in biologic fluid following drug administration during a dosing interval.
pharmacodynamics (PD)	The relationship between drug exposure and pharmacologic response.
pharmacogenetics (PGt)	The study of a gene involved in response to a drug.
pharmacokinetics (PK)	The relationship of time and drug absorption, distribution, metabolism, and excretion.
phase 1 metabolism	Drug metabolizing processes involving oxidation, reduction, or hydrolysis.
phase 2 metabolism	Conjugative drug metabolic processes.
phenotype	An individual's expression of a physical trait or physiologic function due to genetic makeup and environmental and other factors.
poor metabolizer (PM)	In general, an individual with two "reduced–function" or "loss-of-function" alleles relative to a drug-metabolizing enzyme.
prodrug	A drug that requires conversion to an active form.
tau (τ; time)	The dosing interval.

T_{max} (time)	The time of occurrence of the maximum concentration of drug.
ultrarapid metabolizer (UM)	An individual with a "gain-of-function" allele (e.g., overexpression of a metabolic enzyme).
uptake (influx) transporter	A protein that moves drug into cells/tissues.
volume of distribution (V, Vd, V_1, V_{ss}; vol)	A proportionality constant relating the amount of drug in the body to the drug concentration.

Key Equations

$$AUC = \frac{Dose}{CL}$$	Area under the concentration versus time curve, being directly proportional to the dose and inversely proportional to the clearance (CL).
$$C_{ave}^{ss} = \frac{F \cdot Dose}{CL \cdot \tau}$$	The average steady-state drug concentration being directly related to the bioavailability and the dose and inversely related to the clearance and the dosing interval.
$$D_L = C \cdot Vd$$	The loading dose related to a desired concentration and the volume of distribution.
$$D_M = C_{ss} \cdot CL$$	The maintenance dose related to the desired steady-state concentration and the clearance.
$$F = \frac{AUC_{po}}{AUC_{iv}} \cdot \frac{Dose_{iv}}{Dose_{po}} = \frac{\left(\frac{AUC}{Dose}\right)_{po}}{\left(\frac{AUC}{Dose}\right)_{iv}}$$	Absolute bioavailability relating the extent of absorption of an extravascular dose to the intravenous dose.
$$F = fa \cdot ffp$$	Bioavailability related to the fraction of the dose absorbed and the fraction of the dose that escapes first-pass metabolism.
$$F = (ff \cdot fg) \cdot ffp$$	Bioavailability as above with the fraction of the dose absorbed expanded to include the fraction of the dose that avoids gastrointestinal lumen metabolism/degradation and the fraction that avoids gastrointestinal wall metabolism and/or efflux.
$$\tau = \frac{\ln\left(\frac{C_{max}}{C_{min}}\right)}{k_e}$$	Tau, the dosing interval, as a function of the ln quotient of C_{max} and C_{min} and inversely proportional to the elimination rate constant, k_e.
$$t_{1/2} = \frac{0.693 \cdot Vd}{CL}; \ = \frac{0.693}{k_e}$$	The half-life, being directly related to the volume of distribution and inversely related to the clearance; inversely related to the elimination rate constant, k_e.
$\uparrow, \downarrow$	The number of arrows indicates the relative difference in the magnitude of the change.

Introduction

Pharmacokinetics (PK) is the study of the time course of drug absorption, distribution, metabolism, and excretion (ADME), describing how the body handles a given drug. Thus, these processes determine the plasma concentration versus time profile of a given drug. The pharmacologic effect(s) of a given drug are related to that drug interacting with biologic receptors. As it is not possible to easily measure the drug concentration at the site of the receptors, plasma concentrations are related to the effect(s) based on the assumption that there is equilibration between the drug concentration in plasma and that at the site of the receptors. The study of the relationship between the plasma concentrations of a drug and the observed pharmacologic effects is referred to as **pharmacodynamics (PD)**, and it describes how the drug affects the body. The common variable relating pharmacokinetics and pharmacodynamics is the drug concentration; this relationship is depicted in **Figure 2-1**.

The pharmacokinetics of a given drug "drives" the pharmaco-dynamics of that drug in such a way that the drug concentration in the plasma will be in equilibrium with the drug concentration at the receptor site, and responses to the drug, whether therapeutic or toxic, will be a consequence of the drug concentration. The variability in the response to a given drug is due, in part, to the variability in the pharmacokinetics of the drug, although pharmacodynamic vari-ability is typically greater than pharmacokinetic variability. The variability in the pharmacokinetics and pharmacodynamics can be explained, in part, by **pharmacogenetics (PGt)**.

The clinical application of pharmacokinetics is aimed at optimizing drug therapy by designing a **loading dose** (where appropriate) and an initial maintenance regimen, including the maintenance dose and dosing interval, to keep the drug concen-tration within the desired therapeutic range. This is followed by dosage adjustment based on drug concentration determination for drugs that have a narrow therapeutic range. (i.e., the drug concen-trations eliciting a therapeutic effect are close to or overlap those that elicit an adverse effect).

The design of a loading dose is based on the individual's **vol-ume of distribution (Vd)**, which can be influenced, in part, by drug movement into tissues via transporters that are under genetic regulation. Here, a greater Vd will require a higher loading dose to

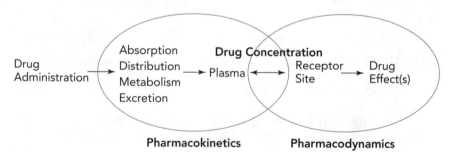

Figure 2-1 The relationship between pharmacokinetics and pharmacodynamics, with the "linking variable" being the drug concentration. As pharmacokinetics determines the plasma concentration versus time profile of the drug, the concentration at the receptor site (i.e., site of action), in equilibrium with the drug in the plasma, elicits the pharmacologic effect(s), which is pharmacodynamics.

achieve a desired drug concentration in the patient. A lesser Vd in a patient would require a lower loading dose. The maintenance dose of a given drug is determined using the drug's **clearance (CL)**. For some drugs, the CL is determined by drug metabolism via specific drug enzymes that also are under genetic regulation. With a greater CL, a higher maintenance dose is required; conversely, a patient with a lower CL would require a lower maintenance dose. The half-life $(t_{1/2})$ of a drug determines its dosing interval. Here, the Vd and CL influence the $t_{1/2}$. With a larger volume of distribution, the drug has to "travel" farther to the eliminating organ for removal from the body. If the CL is held constant, the increased Vd results in a longer $t_{1/2}$ and the drug will remain in the body longer, meaning that the dosing interval, the time to the next dose, will be longer. For a drug that is eliminated from the body by metabolic routes, an increase in CL is related to increased metabolism. This results in a shorter $t_{1/2}$. With a decrease in metabolism, the CL decreases and the $t_{1/2}$ increases. The relationships among Vd, CL, and $t_{1/2}$ are presented in the Key Equations list. Numerous factors influence these relationships, including the patient's genetic constitution. Many of these relationships are discussed further in this chapter.

A number of pharmacokinetic/pharmacodynamic resources describe the mathematical detail of drug-concentration, concentration-effect relationships. The equations in this chapter are presented only to provide a conceptual "framework" of altered pharmacokinetics, here related to PGt.

Absorption and Bioavailability

Oral drug absorption is the process by which a drug moves from the gastrointestinal lumen, crosses biologic membranes, and reaches systemic circulation. With oral administration, the drug travels down the esophagus to the stomach and then to the small intestine. Although some drug can be absorbed from the stomach, it is the small intestine that is the main site of drug absorption. The small intestine's large surface area, permeable membranes, and capillary blood flow create a favorable environment for drug absorption.[1,2]

In order for a drug to be absorbed, it must first be in solution. With oral administration, dissolution of the dosage form, such as a tablet or capsule, results in the drug being in solution in the gastrointestinal lumen, thus creating a concentration gradient of drug across the membranes of the small intestine. This creates a favorable situation for drug absorption, especially via passive diffusion. While passive diffusion is a major mechanism of drug absorption, other absorption mechanisms include active transport, facilitated diffusion (facilitated transport), pinocytosis, and ionic diffusion.[3] When considering mechanisms of absorption, variability in drug absorption has been related to drug transporters, both **uptake (influx) transporters** and **efflux transporters**, which are controlled by the patient's genetic constitution.[4,5]

Oral drug absorption is characterized by the drug's bioavailability, which has clinical relevance. **Bioavailability (F)** can be defined as the rate and extent to which a drug (the active ingredient) is absorbed from a drug product and reaches the general systemic circulation unchanged, being made available to the site of action; that is, once a drug reaches systemic circulation it can be "delivered" to the site of action.[6] As per-oral (po; oral) dosing is the most common route of drug administration, it is the absorption of the drug from the gastrointestinal tract that is of interest and defines oral bioavailability, which will be discussed here. **Figure 2-2** depicts the path a drug takes to reach systemic circulation following oral administration.

The rate of drug absorption is one component of its defined bioavailability. For most clinical purposes, the rate of drug absorption is adequately expressed by the parameter T_{max}. This parameter represents the time of occurrence of the maximum drug concentration following extravascular (e.g., oral) dosing of a drug and is determined by the **absorption rate constant (k_a)** and the **elimination rate constant (k_e)**. The k_a is a rate constant representing the first-order absorption rate of a given drug. The k_e is the rate constant representing the first-order elimination rate of the drug. **Figure 2-3a** presents the concentration versus time profiles of a given drug following oral administration where only the absorption rate constant is altered. **Figure 2-3b** presents the concentration versus time profiles of a given drug following oral administration where only the elimination rate constant is altered for three metabolizer "types" (i.e., poor metabolizer, intermediate metabolizer, extensive metabolizer).

Genetic–Kinetic Interface: T_{max}

An individual may have the genetic constitution that results in the production of an enzyme that is efficient in metabolizing a given drug. In this case, the patient is considered to be an **extensive metabolizer (EM)** of that drug, and the k_e for the drug in this patient is increased relative to that of an **intermediate metabolizer (IM)** or a **poor metabolizer (PM)**. Because the k_e is increased in this individual, indicating that the drug is eliminated faster, the T_{max} will occur sooner. Here, the highest concentration of the drug in this individual will occur sooner rather than later (see Figure 2-3b).

The extent of drug absorption is defined by two parameters: the **maximum concentration (C_{max})** and the area under the drug

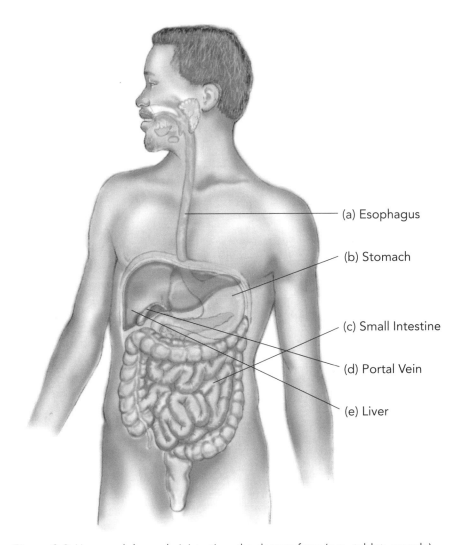

Figure 2-2 Upon oral drug administration, the dosage form (e.g., tablet, capsule) moves down the esophagus (a) to the stomach (b). Although some of the drug may be released from its dosage form and absorbed from the stomach, it is the large surface area of the small intestine (c), with villi and microvilli (not shown), that is the main site of drug absorption. Once drug molecules move across the gastrointestinal wall via various mechanisms, they are carried to the liver (e), via hepatic portal vein blood flow (d), where they may be metabolized. Drug that passes through the liver and reaches systemic circulation is considered to be bioavailable.

concentration versus time curve (AUC_{po}). As a component of bioavailability, the values of these parameters for an orally administered drug are compared to those of the same dose of the drug administered intravenously. Equation 1 describes the calculation of a drug's absolute bioavailability, comparing the **area under the**

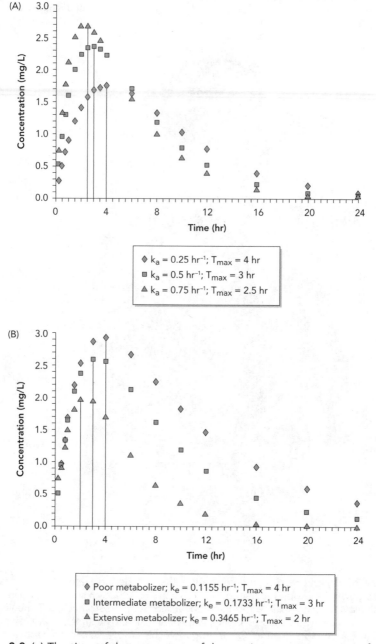

Figure 2-3 (a) The time of the occurrence of the maximum concentration of a drug (T_{max}) is dependent, in part, on the absorption rate constant (k_a). With the elimination rate constant (k_e) fixed, as the k_a increases, the sooner the drug reaches its maximum concentration. The T_{max} is one of the parameters used to describe a drug's bioavailability. (b) The time of the occurrence of the maximum concentration of a drug (T_{max}) is dependent, in part, on the elimination rate constant (k_e). With the absorption rate constant (k_a) fixed, an increased k_e represents increased drug elimination with the maximum concentration being observed earlier (T_{max} occurring sooner). Here, with the examples of a poor metabolizer, intermediate metabolizer, and an extensive (normal) metabolizer. T_{max} is one of the parameters used to describe a drug's bioavailability.

curve (AUC) obtained following oral dosing to that obtained after intravenous dosing:

$$F = \frac{AUC_{po}}{AUC_{iv}} \cdot \frac{Dose_{iv}}{Dose_{po}} = \frac{\left(\dfrac{AUC}{Dose}\right)_{po}}{\left(\dfrac{AUC}{Dose}\right)_{iv}} \qquad (eq. \ 1)$$

Drug administered via the intravenous route is placed directly into systemic circulation, with 100% of the dose reaching systemic circulation, something considered to be "absolute." The ratio of the dose normalized AUC_{po} to the dose normalized AUC_{iv} provides the fraction of the oral dose of the drug that reaches systemic circulation and is termed the absolute bioavailability of the drug and is considered the oral bioavailability.

Genetic–Kinetic Interface: C_{max} and AUC

An individual may have the genetic constitution that results in the production of an enzyme that is inefficient with respect to drug metabolism. In this case, the patient is considered to be a poor metabolizer of that drug, and the C_{max} and AUC for the drug in this patient is increased relative to an intermediate metabolizer or an extensive metabolizer. Such an individual may be at risk of experiencing toxicity, because the drug concentrations will be relatively high (see **Figure 2-4**).

A number of drugs must be "bioactivated" before being able to exert their effects and are administered in the form of a **prodrug**.[7] The bioavailability related to a prodrug points to the active drug reaching systemic circulation. The active drug is formed by metabolic conversion of the "parent" compound. With oral dosing, as the drug moves along the gastrointestinal tract and reaches the small intestine it is presented to and absorbed through the gut wall and then travels to the liver via portal blood flow. Metabolic conversion can take place in the gut wall and/or the liver, with the active drug then reaching systemic circulation. With efficient conversion of the prodrug to the active compound in the gut wall and/or the liver, the active compound will be bioavailable. In the case of inefficient metabolic conversion of a prodrug, more of the parent compound will reach systemic circulation because it will not have been converted to the active compound. **Figure 2-5** shows the concentration versus time profiles for the parent compound and the active compound in an extensive metabolizer and a poor metabolizer.

The bioavailability of a drug is the fraction of the dose that reaches systemic circulation unchanged and is "made available" to the site of action. Conceptually, this fraction is a product of the fraction of the

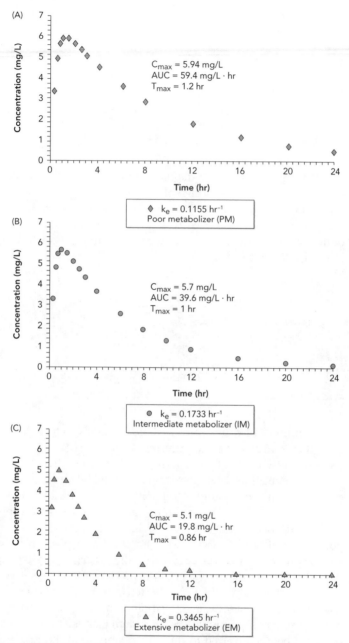

Figure 2-4 As the elimination rate constant (k_e) increases the C_{max} and AUC are lower and the T_{max} occurs earlier. Panel (a) shows the concentration versus time data for a drug that reaches systemic circulation when the k_e is 0.1155 hr^{-1}. The relatively low elimination rate constant may be seen in a poor metabolizer and result in higher drug concentrations. Panels (b) and (c) show the concentration versus time data when the k_e is increased to 0.1733 hr^{-1} and 0.3465 hr^{-1}, respectively, as may be seen in an intermediate metabolizer and an extensive (normal) metabolizer.

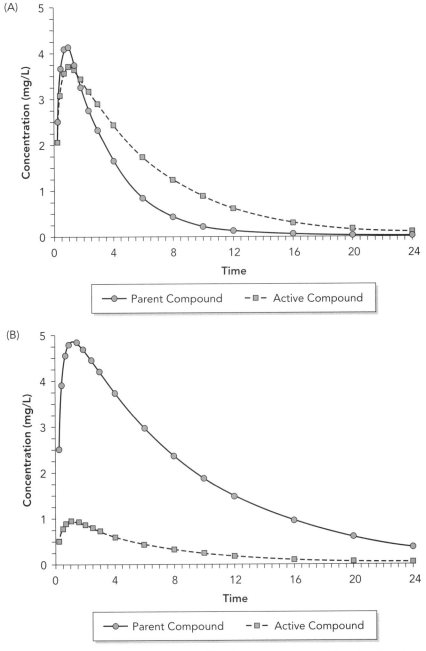

Figure 2-5 Concentration vs. time profile of parent compound (prodrug) and active compound in an extensive metabolizer (EM; panel a) and a poor metabolizer (PM; panel b).

dose of the drug absorbed (fa) and the fraction of the dose of the drug that escapes hepatic first-pass metabolism (ffp; first pass through the liver; Equation 2):

$$F = fa \cdot ffp \qquad \text{(eq. 2)}$$

The fraction of the dose absorbed can further be defined as the fraction of the dose of the drug that is available for absorption (i.e., that which is neither metabolized/degraded in the gastrointestinal lumen nor eliminated in the feces; ff) and the fraction of the dose of the drug that avoids gastrointestinal wall metabolism and/or efflux (fg). Equation 3 defines the bioavailability of a drug as:

$$F = (ff \cdot fg) \cdot ffp \qquad \text{(eq. 3)}$$

Gastrointestinal Wall Influx and Efflux Transporters

Drug molecules that are available for absorption may be "taken up" into intestinal epithelial cells and made available to portal blood flow by influx transporters that serve as a mechanism of drug absorption.[8] Along with other mechanisms of absorption, facilitated transport is recognized as a contributing factor to the bioavailability of some compounds. For instance, a number of organic anion transporting polypeptides (OATP) act as influx transporters.[9] **Table 2-1** lists examples of influx (and efflux) transporters found in the intestinal epithelia that impact drug absorption, thus influencing the bioavailability of drugs that are substrates for such transporters.

Table 2-1

Examples of Gastrointestinal Genes, Transporters, and Drug Substrates

Gene	Transporter/Type	Example Substrates
SLC01A2	OATP/influx	OATP1: enalapril
		OATP2: digoxin, thyroxine, pravastatin
		OATP1/P2: fexofenadine
SLC15A1	PEPT1/influx	β-lactam antibiotics, ACE inhibitors
SLC10A2	ASBT/influx	Benzothiazepine, dimeric bile acid derivatives
SLC16A1	MCT1/influx	Salicylic acid, nicotinic acid
ABCC2	MRP2/efflux	Tamoxifen
ABCG2	BCRP/efflux	Methotrexate, mitoxantrone
ABCB1	P-gp/efflux	Lansoprazole

Genetic–Kinetic Interface: Influx Transporters, F, and $C_{ss,ave}$

An individual may have the genetic constitution that results in the overproduction of a protein that acts to move drug from within the gastrointestinal lumen into the epithelial cells (i.e., an influx transporter). If the drug avoids efflux and/or gastrointestinal epithelial metabolism and escapes first-pass metabolism, the bioavailability will increase for that given drug:

$$\uparrow F = (ff \cdot \uparrow fg) \cdot ffp$$

The increased bioavailability will result in a higher drug concentration (Equation 4):

$$\uparrow C_{ave}^{ss} = \frac{\uparrow F \cdot Dose}{CL \cdot \tau} \qquad \text{(eq. 4)}$$

Here, the individual may be at risk of toxicity as the resultant drug concentration may be too high.

Drug molecules available for absorption may not traverse the gastrointestinal wall because efflux transporters move drug back into the gastrointestinal lumen.[4,5,9,10] These efflux transporters are proteins embedded in the cell membrane that remove drug from the cells. Although these transporters are found on many different cell membranes, the discussion here will focus on the gastrointestinal epithelium.

A number of efflux transporters can impact the bioavailability of a given drug. Two superfamilies of efflux transporters have been studied extensively. These include the adenosine triphosphate (ATP) binding cassette transporters (ABC transporters), which include P-glycoprotein (P-gp), among others, and the solute carrier transporters (SLC transporters).[5,11,12]

As drug in solution crosses the intestinal epithelium, efflux transporters move the drug back to the gastrointestinal lumen. Here, the fraction of the drug that avoids gastrointestinal wall efflux (fg) decreases, and thus bioavailability (F) is decreased. The resultant concentration of the drug in the blood also would be decreased:

$$\downarrow C_{ave}^{ss} = \frac{\downarrow F \cdot Dose}{CL \cdot \tau}$$

Genetic–Kinetic Interface: Efflux Transporters, F, and $C_{ss,ave}$

An individual may have the genetic constitution that results in the overexpression (overproduction) of a protein that acts to move drug from within gastrointestinal epithelium cells back into the gastrointestinal lumen (i.e., an efflux transporter; e.g., P-glycoprotein). In this case, less of the given drug in this patient avoids efflux (fg), and F is decreased:

$$\downarrow F = (ff \cdot \downarrow fg) \cdot ffp$$

The decreased bioavailability will result in a lower drug concentration:

$$\downarrow C_{ave}^{ss} = \frac{\downarrow F \cdot Dose}{CL \cdot \tau}$$

Here, the individual may be at risk of treatment failure because the drug concentrations will be relatively low (i.e., subtherapeutic) (see **Figure 2-6**). The dose of the drug may need to be increased or an alternative drug may need to be used.

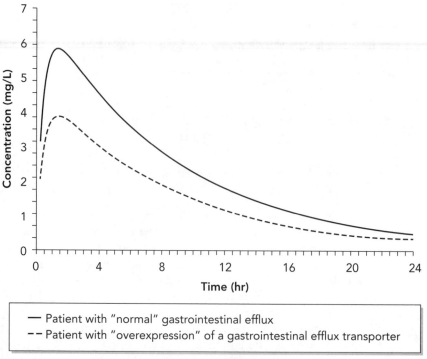

Figure 2-6 Overexpression of an efflux transporter in the gastrointestinal tract results in a decrease in the fraction of the dose that avoids efflux, thus decreasing bioavailability and drug concentration.

Efflux transporters in the gastrointestinal tract can play a major role in the bioavailability of drugs that require transport across the gut wall. Succinctly, with all other processes remaining constant relative to the pharmacokinetics of a drug, "overexpression," or increased activity of gastrointestinal efflux transporters, results in decreased bioavailability and lower systemic drug concentrations, whereas "underexpression," or decreased activity of gastrointestinal efflux transporters, results in increased bioavailability and higher systemic drug concentrations.

Gastrointestinal Wall Metabolism

As drug in solution in the gastrointestinal lumen makes its way into the gastrointestinal epithelium, it may be subject to metabolism by enzymes in the epithelium. Drug metabolized by gastrointestinal wall enzymes does not reach systemic circulation, and thus results in decreased bioavailability; that is, the fraction of the dose avoiding gastrointestinal wall metabolism (f_g) decreases, as does the fraction of the dose that reaches circulation (Equation 3). This, too, will affect the drug concentration. Although there is large interindividual variability in the content of gastrointestinal wall cytochrome P450 isozymes, the average percent content of CYP3A, CYP2C9, CYP2C19, CYP2J2, and CYP2D6 in the gastrointestinal tract is 82%, 14%, 2%, 1.4%, and 0.7%, respectively.[13]

Poor metabolizers would be expected to have more drug avoid gut wall metabolism. Conversely, extensive and ultrarapid metabolizers would be expected to have less drug avoid gut wall metabolism. Not only will less drug reach the portal vein to be carried to the liver, but hepatic metabolism will further affect the amount of drug that reaches systemic circulation. In the case of individuals who are extensive or ultrarapid metabolizers, too little of the drug may be available systemically to be effective, and other therapeutic modalities may be required. **Figure 2-7** shows the relative differences in the concentration versus time data for a poor metabolizer, an intermediate metabolizer, an extensive metabolizer (normal; wild-type), and an ultrarapid metabolizer. With ultrarapid metabolizers, an alternative therapy may be required, because the drug concentration may not achieve therapeutic levels.

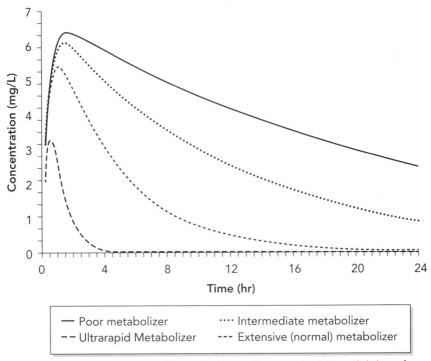

Figure 2-7 Gastrointestinal wall metabolism influences the bioavailability of a given drug. Compared to the extensive (wild type; "normal") metabolizer (EM), the poor metabolizer (PM) exhibits a concentration versus time profile with a T_{max} that occurs later and a C_{max} and AUC that are higher. The intermediate metabolizer (IM) falls between the PM and the EM. The EM and UM have a T_{max} that occurs earlier, and a C_{max} and AUC that are lower, relative to the IM and PM. The bioavailability for a given drug in each individual may be different, due, in part, to genetic (single nucleotide polymorphism) differences between the individuals.

Genetic–Kinetic Interface: Gut Wall Metabolism

An individual may have the genetic constitution that results in CYP2C19 ultrarapid metabolism, (e.g., the *17/*17 genotype). In this case, following per-oral administration of a CYP2C19 substrate drug, less of the drug avoids gastrointestinal wall metabolism (fg), and F is decreased:

$$\downarrow F = (ff \cdot \downarrow fg) \cdot ffp$$

The decreased bioavailability will result in a lower drug concentration:

$$\downarrow C_{ave}^{ss} = \frac{\downarrow F \cdot Dose}{CL \cdot \tau}$$

Here, the individual may be at risk of treatment failure because the drug concentrations will be relatively low. The dose of the drug may need to be increased, or an alternative drug may need to be used.

Hepatic First-Pass Metabolism

Following oral dosing, drug that is available for absorption and that avoids gastrointestinal efflux and gut wall metabolism is carried via hepatic portal blood flow to the liver, where it may be subject to hepatic metabolism, thus undergoing first-pass metabolism. Drug that escapes hepatic metabolism and reaches systemic circulation is said to be bioavailable.

The same potential differences exist for drug metabolism in the liver as were described for gut wall metabolism. Drug that does make it to the liver may be efficiently metabolized in a patient who is an extensive metabolizer or an ultrarapid metabolizer, leaving little drug reaching systemic circulation. Conversely, the patient may be a poor metabolizer with inefficient hepatic metabolism, thus allowing a higher fraction of the drug to reach systemic circulation, resulting in relatively higher bioavailability. The percentage content of cytochrome P450s in the liver has been reported to be 40%, 25%, 18%, 9%, 6%, 2%, and <1%, for CYP3A, CYP2C, CYP1A2, CYP2E1, CYP2A6, CYP2D6, and CYP2B6, respectively.[14]

Genetic–Kinetic Interface: Hepatic First-Pass Metabolism

An individual may have the genetic constitution that results in the under expression of a drug-metabolizing enzyme (e.g., CYP2C19). In this case, more of the given drug in this patient avoids hepatic first-pass metabolism (ffp), and F is increased:

$$\uparrow F = (ff \cdot fg) \cdot \uparrow ffp$$

The increased bioavailability will result in a higher drug concentration:

$$\uparrow C_{ave}^{ss} = \frac{\uparrow F \cdot Dose}{CL \cdot \tau}$$

Here, the individual may be at risk of toxicity because the drug concentration will be relatively high. The dose of the drug may need to be decreased, or an alternative drug may need to be used.

Gastrointestinal Wall Efflux, Metabolism, and Hepatic First-Pass Metabolism

The genetic constitution of an individual will influence each of the variables that determine bioavailability. For instance, a patient may overexpress the efflux transporter protein P-gp while also being an ultrarapid metabolizer who overexpresses CYP2C19. If a drug is subject to efflux by P-gp and is a metabolic substrate for CYP2C19, the bioavailability of that drug would be expected to be quite low because the fraction avoiding efflux, escaping gut wall metabolism, and escaping hepatic first-pass metabolism would be low:

$$\downarrow\downarrow\downarrow F = (ff \cdot \downarrow\downarrow fg) \cdot \downarrow ffp$$

A drug "handled" in this way by the body may not be suitable for oral administration and may need to be administered by a route that avoids gastrointestinal efflux, gastrointestinal wall metabolism, and first-pass metabolism, such as the intravenous or sublingual route, or an alternative drug may need to be used. **Figure 2-8** shows the potential consequences for a drug molecule relative to oral absorption and bioavailability. Recognize that all the potential processes of a given drug's absorption are influenced by the patient's genetic constitution.

Distribution and Volume of Distribution

Influx and efflux transporters are found in many tissues and play a role in the distribution of drugs throughout the body. As discussed previously, transporters in the gastrointestinal epithelium can influence drug absorption and bioavailability. However, these transporters do not influence the distribution of a drug because distribution occurs after the drug reaches systemic circulation. The volume of distribution (Vd) is the proportionality constant relating the amount of drug in the body to the drug concentration.

As traditionally described, the volume of distribution is a primary independent pharmacokinetic parameter that influences the half-life (Equation 5) and is used in the calculation of a drug's loading dose (Equation 6):[15]

$$t_{1/2} = \frac{0.693 \cdot Vd}{CL} \qquad\qquad (eq.\ 5)$$

$$D_L = C \cdot Vd \qquad\qquad (eq.\ 6)$$

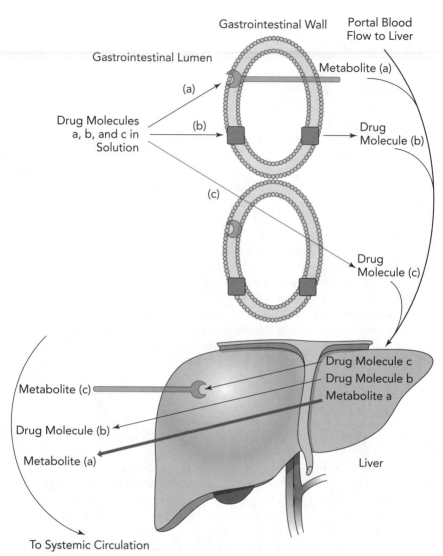

Figure 2-8 Drug being absorbed from the gastrointestinal tract. Upon oral dosing of a given drug, drug molecules a, b, and c, in solution in the gastrointestinal tract, are presented for absorption. Drug molecule (a) is metabolized by an enzyme in the gastrointestinal wall and does not reach systemic circulation and is therefore not bioavailable. The resulting metabolite travels to the liver, via portal blood flow, and then to systemic circulation. Drug molecule (b) is transported, via a protein, from the gastrointestinal lumen to portal blood flow, where it travels to the liver. The molecule moves through the liver and reaches systemic circulation, thus being bioavailable. Drug molecule (c) passively diffuses through the gastrointestinal wall and travels to the liver via portal blood flow. The drug molecule does not reach systemic circulation and is not bioavailable as it is metabolized in the liver (i.e., first-pass metabolism).

Alterations in a drug's volume of distribution can effect the drug's plasma concentration and its efficacy and/or the likelihood of producing toxicity. Rearrangement of Equation 6 shows the implications of an altered volume of distribution relative to the drug concentration:

$$C = \frac{D_L}{Vd} \qquad \text{(eq. 6a)}$$

Equations 5, 6, and 6a represent relationships for a one-compartment pharmacokinetic model where a drug distributes efficiently throughout the body and administration and elimination are into and from a single compartment. This model describes drugs that exhibit a single declining slope on a semi-log plot, following the maximum concentration, when concentrations are observed over time following drug administration.

Following drug administration, many drugs however exhibit more than one declining log-concentration slope over time, suggesting that the drug distributes at different rates into different tissues and that the rate of elimination is slower than the rate of distribution. In this case, the drug concentration versus time data are best described by multi-compartment models. Here, these models describe drug typically administered into the initial volume (V_1), which represents a component of the total volume of distribution (V_{ss}). Ideally, the initial volume of distribution is calculated by dividing the intravenous push (bolus) dose by the initial drug concentration observed immediately after administration of the intravenous push dose. By definition, volumes of a multi-compartment model are additive, thus V_1 (the volume of the first compartment) is smaller than the V_{ss}. Typically, for a multi-compartment model, V_1 is relatively small because immediately after a push dose drug has not yet moved into slowly perfused tissues (i.e., the drug has not equilibrated with other tissue volumes). Also in these models, drug is typically shown to be eliminated from V_1 because the major, "high blood flow" eliminating organs (i.e., kidneys and liver) are considered to be in V_1. Relationships of pharmacokinetic parameters and calculation of the loading dose for a multi-compartment drug as shown in Equations 7 and 7a are related to a multi-compartment model and are similar to the equations for a one-compartment model (Equations 6 and 6a).

$$D_L = C \cdot V_1 \text{ or } D_L = C \cdot V_{ss} \qquad \text{(eq. 7)}$$

$$C = \frac{D_L}{V_1} \text{ or } C = \frac{D_L}{V_{ss}} \qquad \text{(eq. 7a)}$$

For calculation of the loading dose for a drug that has its concentration versus time profile best described by a multi-compartment model, V_1 is used when distribution from the first compartment to the other compartments is relatively slow, whereas V_{ss} is used when distribution from the first compartment to other compartments is relatively rapid.

The distribution of a given drug may depend on the function of a drug transporter such that its overexpression or underexpression alters the volume of distribution, which then may alter the half-life. Additionally, as we have learned more regarding the location and function of certain transporters, it has become clear that in some cases there is a relationship between the volume of distribution and clearance, a measure of drug removal from the body, that may or may not influence the half-life.[16]

As noted earlier, P-gp, an efflux transporter, is expressed in many tissues in the human body, including the liver, kidney, lung tissue, and, to a lesser extent, muscle, mammary glands, and other tissues. As P-gp works to keep drugs out of tissues, underexpression of P-gp would allow for greater distribution of a P-gp substrate drug; the drug would not be removed from the tissue as it would if P-gp were normally expressed. This would increase the volume of distribution of the drug. If the Vd or V_1 (and hence V_{ss}) of the drug were to be the only altered parameter, it would be expected, that the $t_{1/2}$ would be increased also (Equation 5). It also is noted that the calculated loading dose would be higher (Equations 6 and 7). The above scenario implies that the tissue "protected" by P-gp would not serve to metabolize and/or eliminate the given drug, because the volume of distribution was the sole parameter that was altered, with clearance remaining unchanged.[12,16]

Genetic–Kinetic Interface: Drug Distribution, Vd, CL, $t_{1/2}$, and Drug Concentration

An individual with a reduced-function allele for OATP1B1 (resulting in underexpression in liver tissue) is receiving atorvastatin for the treatment of hypercholesterolemia. Atorvastatin is a substrate for OATP1B1 and is metabolized in the liver. The genetic constitution of this individual results in a decreased volume of distribution and a decreased clearance of atorvastatin:

$$\leftrightarrow t_{1/2} = \frac{0.693 \cdot Vd \downarrow}{CL \downarrow}$$

Here, conceptually, it would be expected that the drug concentration would increase because the initial dose is administered into what is effectively a smaller volume of distribution in this individual:

$$\uparrow C = \frac{D_L}{\downarrow Vd}$$

Additionally, as a maintenance dose (D_M) is continued in this individual, the average steady-state concentration will be increased further as the clearance is decreased (Equation 8):

$$D_M = CL \cdot C_{ave}^{ss}$$

(eq. 8)

$$\uparrow C_{ave}^{ss} = \frac{F \cdot Dose}{\downarrow CL \cdot \tau}$$

Although the half-life may not be altered, increases in the drug concentration put the patient at potential risk of toxicity.

Table 2-2

Examples of Overexpression of Drug Transporters in Tissues in Humans and Effects on the Volume of Distribution and the Drug Concentration

Transporter (Type)	Example Tissue	Gene	Effect on Volume of Distribution	Effect on the Plasma Drug Concentration
P-gp (efflux)	Liver	ABCB1	Decrease	Increase
OATP1B1 (influx)	Brain	SLC01B1	Increase	Decrease
OCT1 (influx)	Kidney	SLC22A1	Increase	Decrease

The influx transporter OATP1B1, an organic anion transporter, is expressed in human liver tissue. If a given drug is an uptake substrate for OATP1B1 and also is metabolized in the liver, alterations in the expression of OATP1B1 will have an effect on the volume of distribution and on the clearance of the drug.[17–19] Here, Vd and CL will change in the same direction. The magnitude of change in each parameter will determine whether the $t_{1/2}$ remains constant or is altered (Equation 5). In this situation, clearance is related to the Vd of the drug.

The relationship between Vd and CL can be thought of as a relationship between the physical volume in which the drug resides and the functional mechanism of drug elimination that occurs in that volume.

The genetically controlled tissue expression of a given drug transporter is critical in understanding how a drug's pharmacokinetics are related to the drug concentration. **Table 2-2** shows the tissue distribution of example drug transporters in humans and how genetic variation influences drug distribution and drug concentration.

Metabolism

Many drugs are not excreted from the body unchanged; therefore, they require metabolic conversion to be inactivated and primed for removal via excretory pathways. Genetic variation in the expression and/or activity of drug metabolizing enzymes can have a profound effect on the concentration versus time profiles of these drugs and, more importantly, on the therapeutic outcomes of drug therapy. With two phases of drug metabolism, the potential exists for genetic variability to disrupt drug metabolism, especially for a drug which undergoes each phase of metabolism.

Phase I metabolism refers to chemical reactions involving oxidation, reduction, or hydrolysis. These reactions work to make the drug more polar by adding functional amino, sulfhydral, hydroxyl, and carboxyl groups that make the given drug more hydrophilic, thus promoting excretion of the drug from the body, such as being eliminated in urine.[20] **Phase II metabolism** typically refers to conjugation reactions, including glucuronidation, sulfation, acetylation, and methylation, among other reactions. Phase II metabolism, like phase I metabolism, works to make molecules more water soluble, promoting drug excretion. Both phase I and phase II metabolic reactions are under genetic control, and polymorphisms have been identified for specific enzymes that perform these metabolic functions.

A drug undergoing phase I metabolism may be converted to inactive metabolite(s) that may be excreted or act as substrate(s) for phase II metabolic reactions. Alternatively, a drug may undergo phase I metabolism, resulting in the drug being "activated," which is the premise for the development of prodrugs. Finally, in some cases, the "inactivation" of a drug by phase I and/or phase II metabolism may result in the formation of a toxic metabolite. In this case, the drug is inactivated and no longer produces the desired therapeutic response; however, the metabolite is toxic, eliciting an adverse reaction or unwanted effect.

With respect to phase I oxidative metabolism, the **cytochrome P450 enzyme (CYP)** superfamily has been the focus of extensive research. Although there are numerous CYP enzyme families, three families in particular (CYP1, CYP2, and CYP3) encompass the major drug metabolizing enzymes, with CYP3A being the most prominent.[21] **Table 2-3** presents examples of the CYP enzymes with polymorphisms involved in drug metabolism and the tissues in which these enzymes are expressed. **Figure 2-9** shows the nomenclature for cytochrome P450 enzymes, and **Figure 2-10** presents the contribution of various CYPs in drug metabolism.

Table 2-3

Examples of Cytochrome P450 Drug Metabolizing Enzyme Tissue Expression, Allele Variation, Metabolic Consequence, and Influence on Drug Concentration

CYP Enzyme	Example Tissue Expression	Gene (SNP) rs#[a]	Primary Pharmacokinetic Alteration	Effect on Drug Concentration
CYP2C9	Small intestine/ liver	CYP2C9*2 (C>430>T) rs1799853	Poor metabolizer: increased ffp, decreased CL	Increased fraction of drug dose presented to the liver. Increased concentration.
CYP2C19	Liver	CYP2C19*2 (G>681>A) rs4244285	Poor metabolizer: decreased CL	Increased concentration.
CYP2D6	Liver	CYP2D6*4 (G>1846>A) rs3892097	Poor metabolizer: decreased CL	Increased concentration.

[a] Reference SNP (refSNP) number. These numbers are unique and consistent identifiers of the given SNP.

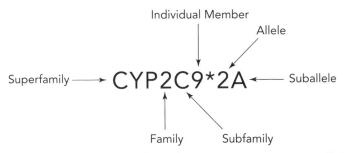

Figure 2-9 Naming nomenclature of cytochrome P450 enzymes. Here CYP2C9*2A is the example CYP enzyme.

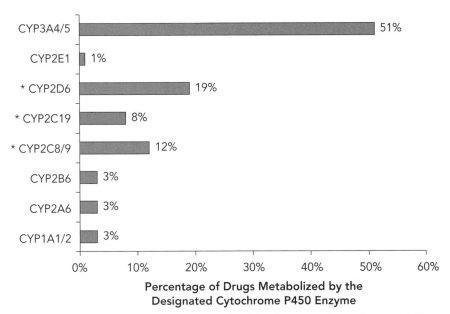

Figure 2-10 Percentage of drugs metabolized by designated cytochrome P450 (CYP) enzymes. Polymorphic (*) expression of certain CYP enzymes confounds the concentration vs. time profile of the drug and may alter the therapeutic response in individuals, thus requiring specific dosing considerations.

Because metabolism of a given drug influences the clearance of that drug and clearance is used to calculate the maintenance dose, identifying a single nucleotide polymorphism (SNP) related to a given CYP enzyme can aid in "personalizing" an individual's dose. Single nucleotide polymorphisms can result in a patient handling a drug in such a manner that they would be considered to be a particular "type" of metabolizer. Homozygous individuals with a polymorphism resulting in the expression of a "loss-of-function" (inactive) or "reduced-function" CYP enzyme would be considered a poor metabolizer. These individuals would have a decreased clearance of substrate drugs and would require a lower maintenance dose to achieve the desired therapeutic response. Individuals who are heterozygous, with one allele producing a loss-of-function or decreased-function enzyme and the other producing a normal-function enzyme, are termed intermediate metabolizers. These individuals may require a lower maintenance dose because they would have a decreased clearance. However, the reduction in clearance would not be as great as that seen in a poor metabolizer, and the required maintenance dose would not be as low. Extensive metabolizers are individuals who have two normal function alleles, and would receive the "normal" maintenance dose. The fourth type of individual would be one in whom there is gene duplication with a consequential overexpression of the CYP enzyme, resulting in a high clearance of the drug, necessitating a higher maintenance dose. These individuals are called **ultrarapid metabolizers (UM)**.

Terminology used to describe the types of phenotypic metabolizers insinuates two concepts related to drug metabolism. The first is the extent of metabolism, and the second is the rate of metabolism. These terms are related to pharmacokinetics in that the phenotypic category of a given individual (i.e., poor metabolizer, intermediate metabolizer, extensive metabolizer, or ultrarapid metabolizer) implies the characteristics of specific pharmacokinetic parameters and dosing requirements. As described above, clearance is the primary pharmacokinetic parameter that is affected by an individual's genetic constitution. This will result in a potential alteration in the half-life because it is dependent on the clearance (and the volume of distribution). Also, an altered clearance will impact the maintenance dose, and the half-life will influence the dosing interval. **Table 2-4** describes the impact of **phenotype** on pharmacokinetic parameters related to metabolism and dosing considerations.

It is important to understand that an individual's **genotype** may not match their phenotype, in that influences other than genetics can alter the expression of a metabolizing enzyme. For instance, an individual with the *1/*1 genotype for CYP2C19 (CYP2C19*1/*1) would be considered an extensive (or "normal") metabolizer. However, if this individual is receiving a certain proton pump inhibitor (PPI), such as omeprazole, for the treatment of esophageal reflux disease, the PPI may inhibit the function of CYP2C19, thus causing the individual to effectively be a poor metabolizer.[22] Here, due to the drug interaction, the individual has the phenotype of a poor metabolizer. It is always important to consider drug–gene interactions and drug–drug interactions simultaneously.

Table 2-4

Metabolic Phenotypes: Pharmacokinetic and Dosing Consequences[a]

Phenotype	Pharmacokinetic Parameter	Consequence	Dosing	Potential Consequence
Poor metabolizer (PM)	k_e; elimination rate constant/$t_{1/2}$; half-life (related to k_e)	↓↓/↑↑	Dosing frequency	↓↓
	CL; clearance	↓↓	Average concentration	↑↑
Intermediate metabolizer (IM)	k_e; elimination rate constant/$t_{1/2}$; half-life (related to k_e)	↓/↑	Dosing frequency	↓
	CL; clearance	↓	Average concentration	↑
Extensive metabolizer (EM)	—	—	—	—
Ultrarapid metabolizer (UM)	k_e; elimination rate constant/$t_{1/2}$; half-life (related to k_e)	↑↑/↓↓	Dosing frequency	↑↑
	CL; clearance	↑↑	Average concentration	↓↓

[a] Relative to the extensive metabolizer being considered "normal," with the same dose being administered to each individual with a given phenotype: ↓ = decreased, ↑ = increased. The number of arrows indicates the relative magnitude of the consequence.

Genetic–Kinetic Interface: Drug Metabolism, CL, Dose, and Dosing Interval

An individual with inheritance of alleles resulting in CYP2D6 gene duplication is receiving doxepin for the treatment of depression. Doxepin, a tricyclic antidepressant, is metabolized by CYP2D6. The genetic constitution of this individual results in the individual being an ultrarapid metabolizer, exhibiting a significantly higher clearance of doxepin. This individual has been taking the drug, but has not been responding. This could be due to the increased clearance of the drug, resulting in low concentrations and drug exposure (Equation 9):

$$\downarrow\downarrow C_{ave}^{ss} = \frac{F \cdot Dose}{\uparrow\uparrow CL \cdot \tau}$$

$$\downarrow\downarrow AUC = \frac{Dose}{\uparrow\uparrow CL} \qquad \text{(eq. 9)}$$

The increased clearance will require an increased maintenance dose to achieve the desired concentration that would maximize the probability of a therapeutic response:

$$\uparrow\uparrow D_M = \uparrow\uparrow CL \cdot C_{ave}^{ss}$$

Additionally, the significantly higher clearance seen in an individual who is an ultrarapid metabolizer will result in a shorter half-life:

$$\downarrow\downarrow t_{1/2} = \frac{0.693 \cdot Vd}{\uparrow\uparrow CL}$$

If the individual is to remain on the drug, the frequency of administration will need to be increased to maintain therapeutic concentrations. The dosing interval **tau (τ)** can be estimated for a rapidly absorbed drug as (Equation 10):

$$\downarrow\downarrow \tau = \frac{\ln\dfrac{C_{max}}{C_{min}}}{\uparrow\uparrow k} \qquad \text{(eq. 10)}$$

or specifically for an intravenous medication (Equation 10a):

$$\downarrow\downarrow \tau = \frac{\ln\dfrac{C_{max}}{C_{min}}}{\uparrow\uparrow k} + t_i \qquad \text{(eq. 10a)}$$

where t_i is the infusion time.

Excretion

As previously mentioned, drug influx and efflux transporters are found in many tissues and play a role in the distribution of drugs throughout the body. Not only do these transporters affect distribution, but they can influence the drug's removal from the body through drug excretion.

The renal excretion of a drug, moving the compound from the blood to the urine, can be a consequence of genetically mediated drug transport.[4,23,24] Renal filtration occurs in the glomerulus, and active secretion occurs in the nephron tubules. Both of these sites are "excretory" because drug is moved from the blood to the urine. Relative to tubular secretion, numerous transporters have been identified in kidney tissue, including P-gp (MDR1), OCT1, OAT1, MRP2, cMOAT, and ENT1, among others. **Table 2-5** presents examples of drug transporters in the kidney and their influence on renal drug handling. Transporter distribution among different populations may explain differences in renal excretion of drugs, and SNPs may further delineate drug removal in given individuals.

Table 2-5

Examples of Renal Drug Transporters Responsible for Urinary Excretion

Example Drug	Example Transporter	Renal Drug Process
Cefamandole[a]	OAT1	Renal tubular excretion
Cimetidine[b]	OAT3	Renal tubular excretion
Acyclovir[b]	OCT1	Renal tubular excretion
Amoxicillin[a]	PEPT1	Renal tubular excretion
Zidovudine[b]	OAT4	Renal tubular reabsorption

[a] Inhibitor of transporter.

[b] Substrate of transporter.

Genetic–Kinetic Interface: Renal Drug Excretion

An individual receiving metformin for treatment of type 2 diabetes may have the genetic constitution that results in the expression of a less active form of the drug transporter OCT1 found on the apical side of the proximal and distal tubules in the kidney. This expression results in decreased uptake of metformin from the plasma, resulting in decreased renal clearance, and hence overall clearance because the clearances are additive (Equation 11):

$$\downarrow CL = \downarrow CL_R + CL_{Other} \hspace{2cm} \text{(eq. 11)}$$

However, OCT1 is also found in liver tissue, and the decreased activity in this tissue results in decreased hepatic uptake of metformin, which may alter the drug effect (pharmacodynamics).

Similar to renal drug excretion, biliary excretion is another mechanism of drug elimination. Efflux transporters (MDR1, MDR3, and others) move drug from the hepatocyte into the biliary canaliculi. The drug/metabolite then is moved to the small intestine, where it may be reabsorbed through enterohepatic cycling or excreted from the body in the feces. Therefore, changes in the level of expression/activity of these transporters within the hepatocytes would be expected to impact biliary drug excretion.

Chapter Summary

The pharmacokinetics of a drug are determined by evaluating the concentration of drug in biologic fluids over time. Drug metabolizing enzymes and drug transporters may influence all aspects of the concentration–time profile, including transporters affecting the volume of distribution, which is used in calculating the loading dose and metabolizing enzymes influencing the clearance, which is used in calculating the maintenance dose. Both the volume of distribution and the clearance influence the elimination rate constant, and hence the half-life, which is used to calculate the dosing interval. It is clear that genetic variation in transporters and metabolizing enzymes are responsible for the varied dosing regimens of the same drug required by different individuals.

Review Questions

1. The study of a gene involved in response to a drug is referred to as:
   a. pharmacokinetics.
   b. pharmacodynamics.
   c. pharmacogenetics.
   d. pharmacogenomics.

2. The _____ is the main site of drug absorption due to its large surface area, membrane permeability, and capillary blood flow.
   a. liver
   b. large intestine
   c. small intestine
   d. stomach

3. If an individual is an extensive metabolizer of a drug relative to an intermediate metabolizer or a poor metabolizer, what happens to the k_e and T_{max} of that drug?
   a. k_e is decreased and the drug is eliminated more slowly; therefore, the T_{max} will occur later.
   b. k_e is decreased and the drug is eliminated faster; therefore, the T_{max} will occur sooner.
   c. k_e is increased and the drug is eliminated more slowly; therefore, the T_{max} will occur later.
   d. k_e is increased and the drug is eliminated faster; therefore, the T_{max} will occur sooner.

4. The _____ of drug absorption is expressed by T_{max}, and the _____ of drug absorption is defined by C_{max} and AUC.
   a. rate; extent
   b. extent; rate
   c. concentration; time
   d. time; concentration

5. With respect to drug metabolism, which individual, relative to metabolizer status, may be at risk of experiencing toxicity from a standard dose of a particular drug (not referring to a prodrug)?
   a. Poor metabolizer
   b. Intermediate metabolizer
   c. Extensive metabolizer
   d. Ultrarapid metabolizer

6. Compared to an extensive metabolizer, an ultrarapid metabolizer will need _____ dosing frequency.
   a. a decreased
   b. an increased
   c. the same
   d. Not enough information has been provided to answer this question.

7. If an individual has a genetic constitution that results in the decreased production of gastrointestinal influx transporters, what will happen to the bioavailability and concentration of a drug that is a substrate for the transporters?
   a. Bioavailability will increase; the concentration will decrease.
   b. Bioavailability will increase; the concentration will increase.
   c. Bioavailability will decrease; the concentration will decrease.
   d. Bioavailability will decrease; the concentration will increase.

8. How might treatment outcome be affected if less of a dose of drug avoids gastrointestinal wall metabolism in a patient?
   a. The patient may be at risk of treatment failure due to low drug concentrations.
   b. The patient may be at risk of toxicity due to high drug concentrations.
   c. The patient may be at risk of treatment failure due to increased bioavailability.
   d. The patient may be at risk of toxicity due to increased bioavailability.

9. _____ or _____ activity of gastrointestinal efflux transporters results in decreased bioavailability and potentially lower systemic drug concentrations.
   a. Underexpression; decreased
   b. Underexpression; increased
   c. Overexpression; decreased
   d. Overexpression; increased

10. With regards to the following equation, if the fraction of a drug that avoids gastrointestinal wall efflux decreases, what would happen to the resultant concentration of the drug in the blood?

$$C_{ave}^{ss} = \frac{F \cdot Dose}{CL \cdot \tau}$$

   a. Decreased
   b. Increased
   c. No change
   d. Not enough information has been provided to answer the question.

11. An individual has the genetic constitution that shows "loss-of-function" of the drug metabolizing enzyme CYP2C19, and this individual is taking a drug that is metabolized by this isozyme. With regards to hepatic first-pass metabolism, _____ of the given drug avoids metabolism, resulting in _____ bioavailability of the drug.
    a. more; increased
    b. more; decreased
    c. less; increased
    d. less; decreased

12. On average, which cytochrome P450 enzyme has the highest percentage of presence in both the gut wall and the liver?
    a. CYP2C9
    b. CYP3A4/5
    c. CYP2C19
    d. CYP2D6

13. An individual overexpresses the efflux protein P-gp and also is an ultrarapid metabolizer, overexpressing CYP2C19. If a drug is a metabolic substrate for CYP2C19 and is subject to efflux by P-gp, what would be the effect on bioavailability? Consider that:

$$F = (ff \cdot fg) \cdot ffp$$

    a. Bioavailability would decrease.
    b. Bioavailability would increase.
    c. Bioavailability would not change.
    d. Not enough information has been provided to answer the question.

14. Influx and efflux transporters in the gastrointestinal epithelium can influence _____ and _____.
    a. distribution of a drug; bioavailability
    b. distribution of a drug; drug absorption
    c. drug absorption; bioavailability
    d. volume of distribution; bioavailability

15. The volume of distribution influences the half-life and is used to calculate a drug's:
    a. maintenance dose.
    b. loading dose.
    c. dosing interval.
    d. a and c

16. _____ is a primary pharmacokinetic parameter that is affected by an individual's genetic constitution.
    a. k_a
    b. $t_{1/2}$
    c. k_e
    d. CL

17. If a patient has underexpression of the influx transporter OATP1B1 in the liver, and the volume of distribution and clearance are decreased by the same magnitude, what change would need to be made to the dosing interval of the drug?
    a. The dosing interval would need to be decreased.
    b. The dosing interval would need to be increased.
    c. The drug would need to be discontinued.
    d. The dosing interval would not need to be changed.

18. A homozygous individual with a polymorphism resulting in a loss-of-function CYP enzyme would be considered a (n) _____ and would have _____ clearance requiring a _____ maintenance dose.
    a. poor metabolizer; increased; higher
    b. extensive metabolizer; increased; higher
    c. poor metabolizer; decreased; lower
    d. extensive metabolizer; decreased; lower

19. An individual with depression has CYP2D6 gene duplication and is considered to be an ultrarapid metabolizer. If this individual is taking the antidepressant doxepin, a CYP2D6 metabolic substrate, what would be the likely treatment outcome and what could be done to correct this?
    a. The individual would likely experience adverse drug reactions due to the relatively high clearance and would require an increased maintenance dose or the use of another drug.
    b. The individual would likely experience adverse drug reactions due to the relatively low clearance and would require a decreased maintenance dose.
    c. The individual would likely experience treatment failure due to the relatively high clearance and would require an increased maintenance dose or the use of another drug.
    d. The individual would likely experience treatment failure due to the decreased clearance and would require a decreased maintenance dose.

20. With regards to renal excretion, if an individual has over-expression of the ABCB1 gene coding for the P-gp (MDR1) transporter in the kidney, what effect would this have on clearance and the drug concentration?
    a. Increased clearance and increased drug concentration.
    b. Decreased clearance and decreased drug concentration.
    c. Increased clearance and decreased drug concentration.
    d. Decreased clearance and increased drug concentration.

References

1. Severijnen R, Bayat N, Bakker H, Tolboom J, Bongaerts G. Enteral drug absorption in patients with short small bowel: A review. Clin Pharmacokinet. 2004;43(14):951–962.

2. Masaoka, Y, Tanaka Y, Kataoka M, Sakuma S, Yamashita S.Site of drug absorption after oral administration: Assessment of membrane permeability and luminal concentration of drugs in each segment of gastrointestinal tract. Eur J Pharm Sci. 2006;29:240–250.

3. Cai1 Z, Wang Y, Zhu L, Liu Z. Nanocarriers: A general strategy for enhancement of oral bioavailability of poorly absorbed or pre-systemically metabolized drugs. Curr Drug Metab. 2010;11:197–207.

4. Kerb R. Implications of genetic polymorphisms in drug transporters for pharmacotherapy. Cancer Lett. 2006;234:4–33.

5. Petzinger E, Geyer J. Drug transporters in pharmacokinetics. N-S Arch Pharmacol. 2006;372:465–475.

6. Guidance for Industry: Bioavailability and bioequivalence studies for orally administered drug products—general considerations. Available at: www.fda.gov/downloads/Drugs/GuidanceComplianceRegulatoryInformation/Guidances/ucm070124.pdf. Accessed September 27, 2011.

7. Rautio J, Kumpulainen H, Heimbach T, et al. Prodrugs: Design and clinical applications. Nat Rev Drug Discov. 2008;7:255–270.

8. Kato Y, Miyazaki T, Sugiura T, Kubo Y, Tsuji A. Involvement of influx and efflux transport systems in gastrointestinal absorption of celiprolol. J Pharm Sci. 2009;98(7):2529–2539.

9. Lan T, Rao A, Haywood J, Davis CB, et al. Interaction of macrolide antibiotics with intestinally expressed human and rat organic anion-transporting polypeptides. Drug Metab Dispos. 2009; 37:2375–2382.

10. Fischer V, Einolf HJ, Cohen D. Efflux transporters and their clinical relevance. Mini-Rev Med Chem. 2005;5:183–195.

11. Chin LW, Kroetz DL. ABCB1 Pharmacogenetics: Progress, pitfalls, and promise. Clin Pharmacol Ther. 2007;81(2):265–269.

12. Cascorbi I. P-glycoprotein: Tissue distribution, substrates, and functional consequences of genetic variations. In: Fromm MF, Kim RB (eds.). Drug transporters: Handbook of experimental pharmacology. Berlin Heidelberg: Springer-Verlag; 2011: 261–283.

13. Paine MF, Hart HL, Ludington SS, Haining RL, Rettie AE, Zeldin DC. The human intestinal cytochrome P450 "Pie." Drug Metab Dispos. 2006;34(5):880–886.

14. Shimada T, Yamazaki H, Mimura M, Inui Y, Guengerich FP. Interindividual variations in human liver cytochrome P-450 enzymes involved in the oxidation of drugs, carcinogens, and toxic chemicals: Studies with liver microsomes of 30 Japanese and 30 Caucasians. J Pharmacol Exp Ther. 1994; 270:414–423.

15. Gibaldi M, Koup JR. Pharmacokinetic concepts: Drug binding, apparent volume of distribution and clearance. Eur J Clin Pharmacol. 1981;20(4):299–305.

16. Grover A, Benet LZ. Effects of drug transporters on volume of distribution. AAPS J. 2009;11(2):250–261.

17. Hagenbuch B, Meier PJ. Organic anion transporting polypeptides of the OATP/ SLCO superfamily, new nomenclature and molecular/functional properties. Pflugers Arch. 2004;447:653–665.

18. Lau YY, Huang Y, Frassetto L, Benet LZ. Effects of OATP1B transporter inhibition on the pharmacokinetics of atorvastatin in healthy volunteers. Clin Pharm Ther. 2007;81:194–204.

19. Chandra1 P, Brouwer KLR. The complexities of hepatic drug transport: Current knowledge and emerging concepts. Pharm Res. 2004;21(5):719–735.

20. Williams DA. Drug metabolism. In: Lemke TL, Williams DA, Roche VF, Zito SW (eds.). Foye's principles of medicinal chemistry. 6th ed. Baltimore, MD: Lippincott Williams & Wilkins; 2008: 253–326.

21. Bartera ZE, Perretta HF, Yeob KR, Allorgec D, Lennarda MS, Rostami-Hodjegan A. Determination of a quantitative relationship between hepatic CYP3A5*1/*3 and CYP3A4 expression for use in the prediction of metabolic clearance in virtual populations. Biopharm Drug Dispos. 2010;31:516–532.

22. O'Donoghue ML. CYP2C19 genotype and proton pump inhibitors inclopido-grel-treated patients. Circulation. 2011;123:468–470.

23. Launay-Vacher V, Izzedine H, Karie S, Hulot JS, Baumelou A, Deray G. Renal tubular drug transporters. Nephron Physiol. 2006;103:97–106.

24. Wolf SJ, Bachtiar M, Wang J, Sim, TS, Chong SS, Lee CGL. An update on ABCB1 pharmacogenetics: Insights from a 3D model into the location and evolutionary conservation of residues corresponding to SNPs associated with drug pharmacokinetics. Pharmacogenomics J. 2011;11:315–325.

Chapter 3

Pharmacogenetics and Pharmacodynamics

LEARNING OBJECTIVES

Upon completion of this chapter, the student will be able to:

1. Recognize the influence of genetic polymorphisms on the efficacy and affinity of drugs.
2. Explain how a specific polymorphism would affect the design of a patient's drug dosing regimen.
3. Differentiate among receptors, enzymes, and transporters as drug targets, and explain how genetic polymorphisms of these drug targets can influence drug selection.
4. Propose alterations to a patient's dosing regimen based on pharmacogenetic influence on pharmacodynamic parameters.

> The student should demonstrate an understanding of how drug targets are influenced by genetic variation. The student should understand that variation in these proteins results in variation in pharmacodynamics, potentially influencing how an individual responds to a given drug.

Key Terms	
affinity	The strength of the reversible binding between a drug and drug target (receptor).
agonist	An endogenous or exogenous ligand that activates a drug target to induce a response.
antagonist	An endogenous or exogenous ligand that inhibits another endogenous or exogenous ligand from binding to a drug target to induce a response.
dissociation constant (K_D)	Describes the ratio of free drug (D) and free receptor (R) concentration to drug–receptor [DR] concentration. Used to determine the affinity of an agonist.
drug resistance	The inability of a drug to produce a pharmacodynamic response at a standard dose.
drug target	Endogenous binding site for drugs. Drug targets can include receptors, enzymes, and membrane transporters.
EC_{50}	The half-maximal (50%) effective concentration of a drug producing a specific response.
efficacy	The effect (E) elicited by a drug (D) and the concentration of drug–receptor complex [DR].
ligand	Endogenous or exogenous agent that binds to a drug target.
pharmacodynamics (PD)	The relationship between drug exposure and pharmacologic response.
potency	The dependence of the pharmacologic effect(s) of the drug on the drug concentration.
serotonin reuptake transporter (SERT)	A transport protein that regulates the amounts of serotonin in the synaptic cleft.

Key Equations	
$Drug\,(D) + Receptor\,(R) \xleftrightarrow[K_2]{K_1} DR\,(response)$	The relationship between free drug concentration (D), free receptor (R) concentration and drug–receptor complex (DR) and drug response.
$K_D = \dfrac{[D][R]}{[DR]}$	Describes the strength of the reversible interaction between a drug and receptor (affinity). K_D is proportional to the free drug concentration and the concentration of unoccupied receptors and is inversely proportional to the drug–receptor complex concentration.

Introduction

The mechanisms of drug action are the fundamental underpinning of pharmacodynamics. Drugs elicit their mechanism(s) of action through biochemical and physiological interactions with drug targets. Thus, the pharmacodynamic effects of a drug determine its overall therapeutic utility. **Pharmacodynamics (PD)** is the relationship between drug exposure and pharmacologic response, with elicited effects being related to drug binding to target proteins such as receptors, enzymes, and membrane transporters. Drugs bind to these targets through a combination of chemical bonding interactions, such as covalent, hydrogen, hydrophobic, ionic, and van der Waals. Because these **drug targets** are all proteins, they are susceptible to the effects of single nucleotide polymorphisms (SNPs). Single nucleotide polymorphisms in the DNA encoding these proteins can result in reduced drug binding (e.g., decreased ability for chemical bonding interactions) and subsequently induce **drug resistance**. Drug resistance is the inability of a drug to produce a pharmacodynamic response at a standard dose. Therefore, the ability to detect SNPs in drug targets represents a method for improving the therapeutic response to drugs.

The **affinity** of a drug for a drug target, such as a receptor, is measured by the strength of the interaction between the drug and the target. The relationship between a drug (D) and receptor (R) determines the drug's overall affinity and efficacy. Affinity describes the strength of the reversible interaction between a drug and drug target. This interaction is described in the following equation:

$$\text{Drug (D)} + \text{Receptor (R)} \underset{K_2}{\overset{K_1}{\longleftrightarrow}} \text{DR (response)} \qquad \text{(eq. 1)}$$

In this equation (Equation 1), the effect (response) of a drug is directly dependent on the DR interaction. Therefore, the ratio of K_2 to K_1, or the dissociation of the drug from the receptor, determines the overall effect of the drug. This ratio (K_2/K_1) is known as the **dissociation constant (K_D)**:

$$K_D = \frac{[D][R]}{[DR]} \qquad \text{(eq. 2)}$$

A high affinity of a drug for a receptor means a small K_D. The generation of a response from the DR complex is determined by the drug's **efficacy**. Efficacy describes the effect (E) elicited by a drug (D) and the concentration of the drug–receptor complex [DR]. Efficacy is a measure of the relative **potency**, or likelihood of a drug to induce a response. Thus, the potency of a drug is determined by the affinity and efficacy of a drug at the receptor. The potency of a drug is also influenced by receptor density and responsiveness at the target tissue.

Genetic–Dynamic Interface: K_D

An individual may have the genetic constitution that results in the reduced expression of a receptor (R). In this case, the patient is considered to be drug resistant. As the concentration of drug–receptor complex [DR] decreases, the concentration of free drug [D] increases, and the overall KD increases (therefore the numerator is increasing while the denominator is decreasing in Equation 2). An increase in K_D means a lower affinity of a drug for a receptor, and the patient could appear to be resistant to the drug's effects.

In general, as the concentration of a drug increases, so does the pharmacologic response. Plotting the magnitude of response against the dose of the drug generates a dose–response curve, as depicted in **Figure 3-1**. Note that the x-axis is the log drug concentration [drug]. Semilogarithmic plots allow for graphing of doses that may span

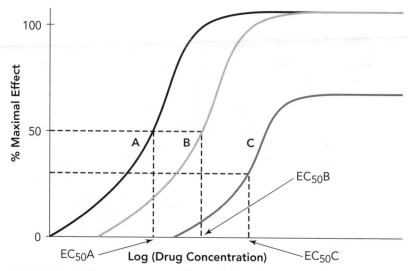

Figure 3-1 Classic dose-response curves. Based on the EC_{50}, the potency of the drugs are in the following order A > B > C. However, drugs A and B have the same efficacy because both reach the same E_{max}. Drug C is less efficacious than both drugs A and B.

several orders of magnitude. Once the maximal drug–receptor complex [DR] concentration is reached, a 100% maximal effect (E_{max}) is achieved, and the dose–response curve plateaus. The drug concentration [D] that produces a 50% maximal response is designated as the effective concentration 50% (**EC_{50}**). The lower the EC_{50} for a drug, the more potent the drug.

Genetic–Dynamic Interface: Dose–Response Curves (Agonist Example)

An individual may have the genetic constitution that results in a heterozygotic genotype, resulting in decreased drug affinity for a given receptor. If curve A in Figure 3-1 is a consequence of the normal expression of the receptor, then curve B could represent an individual who displays a heterozygotic genotype resulting in decreased drug potency ($\uparrow EC_{50}$). In this example, the drug's overall efficacy (E_{max}) did not change. However, a heterozygotic and/or homozygotic genotype of the same receptor could induce the response depicted in curve C; resulting in a decrease in both potency ($\uparrow EC_{50}$) and efficacy ($\downarrow E_{max}$).

Drugs that block the ability of the endogenous **ligand** to bind to the receptor are classified as **antagonists**. In the classic dose–response curves (Figure 3-1), a competitive antagonist shifts the curve to the right (shifting curve A toward curve B). With competitive antagonism, the effects of the antagonist can be reversed by adding sufficient concentrations of agonist. By comparison, noncompetitive antagonism cannot be reversed by adding high concentrations of agonist (shifting curve A toward curve C).

Pharmacogenetics and Receptors as Drug Targets

Endogenous receptor ligands bind to a receptor to stimulate a biochemical and physiological response. For example, during the fight-or-flight response invoked by the activation of the sympathetic nervous system, epinephrine is released in order to activate a cascade of physiologic effects. The epinephrine that is released binds to β_2-adrenergic receptors (β_2AR) in the bronchiolar smooth muscle to induce bronchodilation and increase oxygen exchange, which is required during the fight-or-flight response. In this example, epinephrine is serving as the endogenous ligand, activating β_2-adrenergic receptors as an **agonist**. The β_2-adrenergic receptor is a cell-surface receptor composed of 413 amino acid residues (see **Figure 3-2**). These amino acids are arranged in such a way that the receptor contains seven transmembrane-spanning domains with an extracellular N-terminus and an intracellular carboxy terminus. To date, 49 SNPs have been reported in the β_2-adrenergic

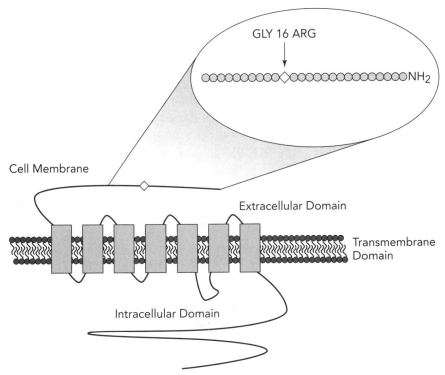

Figure 3-2 The β_2-adrenergic receptor is composed of 413 amino acids. The Gly16Arg amino acid change in the receptor (indicated by the diamond) predisposes patients to nocturnal asthma and influences asthma severity. Note that this amino acid switch occurs in the external-binding domain.

receptor. Five of these have been associated with nonsynonymous (missense) polymorphisms resulting in a change in the amino acid sequence: Ser220Cys, Thr164Ile, Val34Met, Gln27Glu, and Gly16Arg.[1] The Gly16Arg amino acid change in the receptor (protein) predisposes patients to nocturnal asthma and influences asthma severity.[2]

With respect to pharmacodynamics, nonsynonymous SNPs encoding for either Arg or Gly at position 16 have been linked to altered responses to short-acting β_2AR agonists, such as albuterol (Gly at position 16 imparts a better response than Arg at position 16).[1]

Pharmacogenetics and Enzymes as Drug Targets

Enzymes also serve as pharmacodynamic targets for drugs. Like receptor targets, enzymes are composed of amino acids that not only regulate the enzyme's endogenous activity but also the ability of the drug to bind to the enzyme to produce a pharmacodynamic response. Asthma is characterized by increased responsiveness of the tracheobronchial tree to a multiplicity of stimuli. The cysteinyl leukotrienes (LTC4, LTD4, and LTE4) serve as a stimulus to increase bronchiolar smooth muscle contraction and mucus secretion, triggering an asthmatic response. 5-lipoxygenase is an enzyme essential to the biosynthesis of cysteinyl leukotrienes, and it serves as the pharmacodynamic target for drugs such as zileuton (see **Figure 3-3**). By inhibiting 5-lipoxygenase, zileuton decreases the synthesis of cysteinyl leukotrienes, and therefore provides symptomatic relief for the asthma patient.[3] Polymorphisms in the 5-lipoxygenase gene promoter region are associated with differential responses to 5-lipoxygenase inhibitors.[4] Insertion- or deletion-type mutations have been identified in the promoter region of the gene in 22% of Caucasians.

Genetic–Dynamic Interface: 5-Lipoxygenase

Genetic information received through a saliva sample obtained from a patient reveals a deletion polymorphism within the promoter region of the 5-lipoxygenase gene. This deletion results in an altered amino acid sequence within the binding region of the enzyme and decreased zileuton binding to the enzyme. The following inhibitory E_{max} model best describes the altered binding of zileuton:

$$E = E_0 - \frac{(E_{max})(C)}{EC_{50} + C}$$

In this example, the deletion polymorphism within the promoter region results in an increased EC_{50}, and therefore an overall decrease in the patient's sensitivity to zileuton. In this scenario, the patient would require a dose of zileuton that is higher than the standard dose.

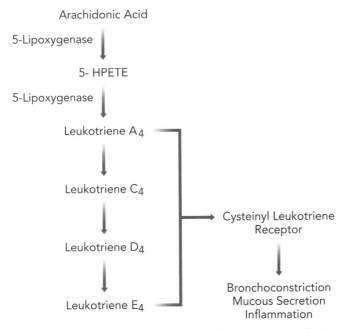

Figure 3-3 The role of 5-lipoxygenase in cysteinyl leukotriene synthesis. The 5-lipoxygenase enzyme catalyzes the initial steps in the synthesis of the cysteinyl leukotrienes LTA4, LTC4, LTD4, and LTE4. These leukotrienes mediate bronchoconstriction, mucous secretion, and the recruitment of inflammatory cell mediators through the activation of the cysteinyl leukotriene receptor. 5-HPETE = 5-Hydroperoxyeicosatetraenoic acid.

Pharmacogenetics and Membrane Transporters as Drug Targets

The termination of neurotransmitter effects in the central nervous system predominantly occurs as a result of neurotransmitter reuptake into the secreting neuron. For example, serotonin is released into the synaptic cleft to activate postsynaptic receptors, inducing a physiologic response (see **Figure 3-4**). Serotonin's effects are terminated in large part by reuptake mediated by the **serotonin reuptake transporter (SERT)**. Once taken back up by the neuron, the serotonin is recycled for later use. The selective serotonin reuptake inhibitors (SSRIs), such as fluoxetine, induce their pharmacodynamic effects through the inhibition of SERT. Inhibition of SERT increases serotonin levels in the synaptic cleft, thereby enhancing serotonin-mediated effects. A polymorphism in the promotor region of the SERT gene has been identified.[5] This polymorphism is often referred to as SERTPR, in reference to the promotor region. Two forms of polymorphisms

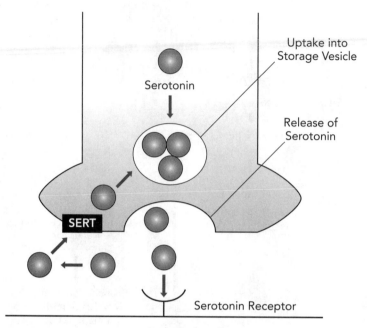

Uptake into
Storage Vesicle

Serotonin

Release of
Serotonin

SERT

Serotonin Receptor

Intracellular Response

Figure 3-4 Serotonin released into the synapse is recycled back into the neuron for later release and use. The reuptake of serotonin into the sertonergic terminal is mediated by the serotonin reuptake transporter (SERT).

have been identified in the SERTPR: long (l) and short (s). Depressed patients who are homozygotic (l/l) or heterozygotic (l/s) for the variant have demonstrated a better response to SSRIs than those homozygotic (s/s) for the short variant.[6] Subsequently, other indications for SSRIs (e.g., anxiety) have also demonstrated similar variations in responsiveness.[7]

Pharmacogenetics and Pharmacodynamics Application

DC is a 29-year-old African American male who presents to his primary care physician's office for initial evaluation in the pharmacotherapy clinic. Today, DC reports wheezing, coughing, and shortness of breath at rest and during activity. DC states he has a history of coughing and wheezing beginning in his teenage years and has been treated for multiple episodes of bronchitis. DC reports that he has had numerous unscheduled doctor visits in the last year, about 15 emergency department visits in the past five years, and that he has been hospitalized seven times in his lifetime, with the last hospitalization being four months ago. DC also complains that he has difficulty exercising and doing some daily activities. DC states that most recently he is feeling short of breath, has a runny nose/nasal congestion, wheezes a few times a week, has night-time symptoms of coughing, and is using his albuterol inhaler daily. His current medications include: albuterol inhaler, two puffs as needed (patient states he has been using it three to four times daily with no relief); Claritin 10 mg, once daily; and Flonase, two inhalations each nostril, as needed.

DC states that he lives alone. His dog sometimes sleeps in the same bed with him; he also has one cat. Carpeting is present throughout his house except for the kitchen and the bathrooms.

With pharmacogenetic testing, DC is found to be homozygous for the SNP that results in the Gly16Arg amino acid sequence change in the β_2 receptor. As stated, his asthma pharmacotherapy consists of a short-acting β_2-agonist, albuterol, which is not providing relief, indicating uncontrolled asthma. Because of the patient's nonsynonymous (homozygotic) SNP resulting in the amino acid change at position 16, he is not responding to his albuterol. Based on the fact that he is frequently self-dosing to no avail, adding an alternative treatment may be of benefit. Two alternatives with different pharmacologic mechanisms to consider would be the addition of a low-dose inhaled corticosteroid or a mast cell stabilizer, such as cromolyn sodium. Additionally, DC should be counseled on the proper use of his medications as well as lifestyle modifications, including no longer allowing his dog to sleep in his bed. Additionally, DC should consider removing the carpeting from his house.

Note that in cases where the patient is homozygotic, switching to an alternative drug with a different mechanism of action may be warranted. In cases where the patient is heterozygotic, increasing the dose may provide a therapeutic response. If it does not, it would be prudent to switch the drug choice to a compound from an alternative pharmacologic class.

Chapter Summary

Pharmacodynamic variability is usually greater than pharmacokinetic variability. The variability results in different responses among patients, related to efficacy and/or toxicity. Here, differences in drug receptors based on an individual's genetic constitution can have a significant influence on whether a patient will respond to a given drug therapy. This represents a genetic–dynamic interaction. In the case where genetic constitution results in a kinetic variance that alters the drug concentration, resulting in a varied clinical effect, we have a genetic–kinetic–dynamic interaction.

Review Questions

1. The study of the relationship between the plasma concentration of a drug and the observed pharmacologic effects is referred to as:
   a. pharmacokinetics.
   b. pharmacodynamics.
   c. pharmacogenetics.
   d. pharmacogenomics.

2. If curve A in the following figure represents the dose–response curve to an agonist, which curve would represent the addition of a noncompetitive antagonist?

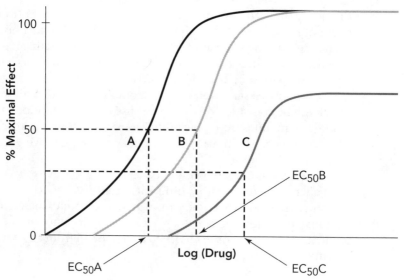

   a. Curve A
   b. Curve B
   c. Curve C

3. If curve B in the following figure represents the dose–response curve of an agonist, which curve would represent the addition of a competitive antagonist in a patient who is homozygotic for a SNP resulting in a conformational change in the receptor so the antagonist cannot be overcome?

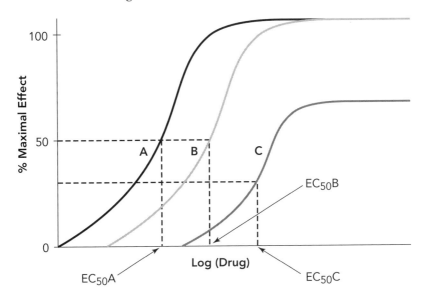

a. Curve A
b. Curve B
c. Curve C

4. An increase in K_D:
   a. results in a lower affinity of a drug for a receptor.
   b. means that a patient could appear to be resistant to the effect of the drug.
   c. could result from a heterozygotic SNP coding for a receptor with decreased drug affinity.
   d. All of the above

5. A SNP that ultimately results in an increased EC_{50} produces:
   a. an overall increase in drug sensitivity.
   b. an overall decrease in drug sensitivity.
   c. no change in drug sensitivity.

References

1. Tatlor MR. Pharmacogenetics of the human beta-adrenergic receptors. *Pharmacogenomics J.* 2007;7(1):29–37.

2. Portelli M, Sayer I. Genetic basis for personalized medicine in asthma. *Expert Rev Respir Med.* 2012;6:223–236.

3. Asano K, Ishizaka A. Pharmacogenetics of anti-leukotriene drugs. *Clin Exp Allergy Rev.* 2008;8:45–49.

4. In KH, Asano K, Beier D, et al. Naturally occurring mutations in the human 5-lipoxygenase gene promoter that modify transcription factor binding and reporter gene transcription. *J Clin Invest.* 1997;99:1130–1137.

5. Heils A, Teufel A, Petri S, et al. Allelic variation of human serotonin transporter gene expression. *J Neurochem.* 1996;66:2621–2624.

6. Serretti A, Benedetti F, Zanardi R, Smeraldi E. The influence of serotonin transporter promoter polymorphisms of the serotonin pathway on the efficacy of antidepressant treatments. *Prog Neuro-Psychopharm Bio Psych.* 2005;29:1074–1084.

7. Stein MB, Seedat S, Gelernter J. Serotonin transporter gene promoter polymorphism predicts SSRI response in generalized social anxiety disorder. *Psychopharmacol.* 2006;187:68–72.

Section **III**

Individual Drugs

Section III presents examples of drugs that have their pharmacokinetics and/or pharmacodynamics influenced by genetics. Examples of pharmacogenetic–pharmacokinetic, pharmacogenetic–pharmacodynamic, and pharmacogenetic–pharmacokinetic–pharmacodynamic interactions are presented. Pharmacogenetic–pharmacokinetic and/or pharmacogenetic–pharmacodynamic interfaces are presented to make clear the influence of genetics on the way the body handles a drug and the way a drug affects the body.

Chapter **4**

Abacavir

LEARNING OBJECTIVES

Upon completion of this chapter, the student will be able to:

1. Recognize the genotype related to abacavir hypersensitivity reaction.
2. Explain the appropriate use of genetic testing in an individual who is to receive abacavir.
3. Interpret and utilize genetic testing information relative to abacavir.

> The student should understand the potential for a gene–drug interaction related to adverse events. The student also should understand that a valid genetic test can identify patients at risk of a severe adverse event, with a potential actionable response being utilization of an alternative drug therapy.

CASE QUESTIONS

Upon completion of this chapter, the student will be able to answer the following questions pertaining to the case of OM:

1. Would genetic testing for the HLA-B*57:01 allele be warranted in OM?
2. What is the proper use of genetic information related to HLA-B*57:01?

Key Terms	
pharmacodynamic	The relationship between drug exposure and pharmacologic response.

Introduction

OM is a 37-year-old Caucasian male with a six-week history of muscle soreness, swollen lymph nodes in the neck, and night sweats and a three week history of a slight rash, with small dark raised bumps on his abdomen and back. He also is experiencing gastrointestinal discomfort and right-lower-quadrant pain.

OM has a history of intravenous narcotic drug abuse, and it has been documented that OM has shared needles with other individuals. Laboratory tests indicate a positive HIV-antigen test, as well as a CD4 count of 372 cells/mm^3. Upon further testing, it is determined that OM is positive for the human immunodeficiency virus (HIV), which is confirmed by the results of a Western blot test. The gastrointestinal symptoms are diagnosed as related neutropenic enterocolitis, a condition well documented as being associated with HIV infection.[1]

Being HIV positive, OM is started on Trizivir, which contains abacavir sulfate (300 mg), lamivudine (150 mg), and zidovudine (300 mg) twice a day. Three weeks after initiation of the triple-drug combination, OM presents to the emergency department with nausea, diarrhea, mild rash, headache, fever, and other constitutional symptoms, including severe fatigue and myalgia.[2,3] Although the symptoms appear to be similar to his original presentation prior to the HIV diagnosis, OM states that the current symptoms seem to "get worse" after each dose of his HIV medication. Additionally, the symptoms continue to become more severe as time progresses. With this information, OM is diagnosed with abacavir hypersensitivity reaction.

A clinical team member wants to perform a challenge test with abacavir using the abacavir "patch test," where a low concentration abacavir gel is prepared and placed on the middle of the back to look for a skin reaction in the subsequent 48 to 72 hours. Redness and swelling would be an indication of hypersensitivity to abacavir.[4] The patch test is not recommended; therefore, it is suggested that genetic testing be utilized to determine if OM expresses the HLA-B*57:01 allele.[5] Studies have shown that individuals with the HLA-B*57:01 allele are at risk of abacavir hypersensitivity reaction.[6–10] The test results in fact show that OM expresses the HLA-B*57:01 allele, strengthening the diagnosis of abacavir hypersensitivity reaction. OM is in the population of U.S. Caucasian patients, in which 7–8% carry the HLA-B*57:01 allele. The frequency of the HLA-B*57:01 allele in the U.S. African American, Hispanic, and Asian populations is 2.5%, 2%, and 1%, respectively.

Abacavir Pharmacodynamics

The influence of genetics relative to abacavir is in reference to a **pharmacodynamic**-mediated allergic response that can result in symptoms that represent delayed hypersensitivity. The mechanism of abacavir hypersensitivity is based on the hapten model, where abacavir is taken up into the cytoplasm of antigen-presenting cells (i.e., cells presenting HLA-B*57:01).[11] Once in the cytosol, abacavir is converted to carbovir and, with the addition of phosphates via kinases, it becomes the active compound carbovir-triphosphate.[11] The triphosphate compound binds to a cytosolic protein resulting in a carbovir–protein conjugate that is presented specifically by HLA-B*57:01 to CD8(+) T-lymphocytes. This specificity is due to the conformation of the carbovir–protein conjugate that results in preferential binding to HLA-B*57:01 for presentation.[11,12] Because the binding is specific for HLA-B*57:01, individuals who express this antigen are at risk for the consequences of T-cell mediated toxicity. This toxicity is mediated by abacavir-specific CD8(+) T-lymphocytes, which secrete interferon-gamma (IFN-γ) and tumor necrosis factor-alpha (TNF-α). Interferon-gamma has been shown to up-regulate HLA presentation; therefore, it may increase the response of CD8(+) T-lymphocytes. Tumor necrosis factor-alpha has been shown to mediate fever, sepsis, and organ failure.[13]

Abacavir hypersensitivity reaction may result in injury to multiple organs, causing a broad range of signs and symptoms. These typically include fatigue, malaise, and myalgia as the most consistent presenting constitutional symptoms. Fever, rash, respiratory, and gastrointestinal signs and symptoms may also be present. Symptoms may appear similar to those seen in patients with influenza A; however, patients with abacavir hypersensitivity have more gastrointestinal signs and symptoms, whereas patients with influenza A have more respiratory signs and symptoms.[3] The rechallenge of a patient with abacavir may result in bronchoconstriction, hypotension, and resultant renal failure. These severe reactions with abacavir rechallenge occur in up to 20% of patients; therefore, abacavir rechallenge is not appropriate.[2,14,15]

Guidelines for HLA-B*57:01 relative to abacavir dosing were presented by the Clinical Pharmacogenetics Implementation Consortium in April of 2012. The consortium strongly recommends that due to the increased risk of abacavir hypersensitivity reaction that abacavir be avoided in patients who express HLA-B*57:01. The recommendations are similar to those of the U.S. Department of Health and Human Services (DHHS) panel on Antiretroviral Guidelines for Adults and Adolescents.[5,16]

Genetic–Dynamic Interface: Abacavir Toxicity

Abacavir toxicity, with respect to hypersensitivity, is related to the HLA-B*5701 allele. The frequency of the HLA-B*5701 allele is dependent on the specific population. The relatively high frequency of the allele in Caucasian populations (7–8%) warrants pharmacogenetic testing prior to the use of abacavir. A Black Box Warning has been added to the package labeling for the drug.[6] It states:

Serious and sometimes fatal hypersensitivity reactions have been associated with ZIAGEN (abacavir sulfate).

Hypersensitivity to abacavir is a multiorgan clinical syndrome usually characterized by a sign or symptom in two or more of the following groups: (1) fever, (2) rash, (3) gastrointestinal (including nausea, vomiting, diarrhea, or abdominal pain), (4) constitutional (including generalized malaise, fatigue, or achiness), and (5) respiratory (including dyspnea, cough, or pharyngitis). Discontinue ZIAGEN as soon as a hypersensitivity reaction is suspected.

Patients who carry the HLA-B*5701 allele are at high risk for experiencing a hypersensitivity reaction to abacavir. Prior to initiating therapy with abacavir, screening for the HLA-B*5701 allele is recommended; this approach has been found to decrease the risk of hypersensitivity reaction. Screening is also recommended prior to reinitiation of abacavir in patients of unknown HLA-B*5701 status who have previously tolerated abacavir. HLA-B*5701-negative patients may develop a suspected hypersensitivity reaction to abacavir; however, this occurs significantly less frequently than in HLA-B*5701-positive patients.

Regardless of HLA-B*5701 status, permanently discontinue ZIAGEN if hypersensitivity cannot be ruled out, even when other diagnoses are possible.

Following a hypersensitivity reaction to abacavir, NEVER restart ZIAGEN or any other abacavir-containing product because more severe symptoms can occur within hours and may include life-threatening hypotension and death.

Reintroduction of ZIAGEN or any other abacavir-containing product, even in patients who have no identified history or unrecognized symptoms of hypersensitivity to abacavir therapy, can result in serious or fatal hypersensitivity reactions. Such reactions can occur within hours.

Lactic acidosis and severe hepatomegaly with steatosis, including fatal cases, have been reported with the use of nucleoside analogues alone or in combination, including ZIAGEN and other antiretrovirals.

Chapter Summary

The status of a patient relative to HLA-B*57:01 imparts a clear approach to antiretroviral therapy with regard to abacavir. Clearly, a patient who expresses HLA-B*57:01 should not receive abacavir, and alternative antiretroviral therapy must be employed.

Answers to Case Questions

1. Diagnosis of abacavir hypersensitivity, through symptoms and timing of therapy, was enough to give reason for discontinuing the drug, and genetic testing would not necessarily be warranted. However, at the time of diagnosis of the HIV infection, if abacavir was being considered for this Caucasian male, testing would be warranted.
2. Because the main issue regarding abacavir use is related to an adverse event, the use of HLA-B*57:01 genetic screening should be considered in the context of safety and prevention. The U.S. DHHS panel on Antiretroviral Guidelines for Adults and Adolescents and the Clinical Pharmacogenetic Implementation Consortium, among others, recommends performing genetic screening for HLA-B*57:01 before starting any abacavir-naïve patient on an abacavir-containing regimen, such as Ziagen and Trizivir.

Review Questions

1. Abacavir toxicity, expressed as a multi-organ clinical syndrome, has been related to which of the following?
   a. HLA-B*15:02
   b. HLA-B*57:01
   c. CYP2C9*1/*1
   d. HLA-A*21:46

2. Which of the following populations are most at risk for a hypersensitivity reaction when prescribed abacavir?
   a. Caucasians
   b. Japanese
   c. Indian
   d. a and c
   e. All of the above are equally at risk.

3. If a patient is suspected of having a hypersensitivity reaction to abacavir, the patient should be challenged with a subsequent dose.
   a. True
   b. False

4. The relationship between abacavir and the genetic constitution of an individual with regard to HLA allele status is an example of a:
   a. genetic–dynamic relationship.
   b. genetic–genomic relationship.
   c. genetic–kinetic relationship.
   d. genetic–metabolic relationship.

5. Based on the Black Box Warning, screening for HLA-B*57:01 is recommended prior to initiating therapy with abacavir.
   a. True
   b. False

References

1. Bavaro MF. Neutropenic enterocolitis. Curr Gastroenter Rep. 2002;4:297–301.
2. Hetherington S, McGuirk S, Powell G, et al. Hypersensitivity reactions during therapy with the nucleoside reverse transcriptase inhibitor abacavir. Clin Ther. 2001;23:1603–1614.
3. Keiser P, Nassar N, Skiest D, et al. Comparison of symptoms of influenza A with abacavir-associated hypersensitivity reaction. Int J STD AIDS. 2003;14:478–481.
4. Phillips EJ, Sullivan JR, Knowles SR, Shear NH. Utility of patch testing in patients with hypersensitivity syndromes associated with abacavir. AIDS. 2002;16:2223–2225.
5. Panel on Antiretroviral Guidelines for Adults and Adolescents. Guidelines for the use of antiretroviral agents in HIV-1-infected adults and adolescents. Washington, DC: U.S. Department of Health and Human Services; 2011: 1–166.
6. Ziagen (abacavir sulfate) prescribing information. Available at: http://us.gsk .com/products/assets/us_ziagen.pdf. Accessed January 16, 2012.
7. Rauch A, Nolan D, Martin A, McKinnon E, Almeida C, Mallal S. Prospective genetic screening decreases the incidence of abacavir hypersensitivity reactions in the Western Australian HIV cohort study. Clin Infect Dis. 2006;43:99–102.
8. Mallal S, Phillips E, Carosi G, et al; PREDICT-1 Study Team. HLA-B*5701 screening for hypersensitivity to abacavir. N Engl J Med. 2008;358:568–579.
9. Hughes AR, Spreen WR, Mosteller M, et al. Pharmacogenetics of hypersensitivity to abacavir: from PGx hypothesis to confirmation to clinical utility. Pharmacogenet J. 2008;8:365–374.
10. Phillips E, Mallal S. Successful translation of pharmacogenetics into the clinic. Mol Diag Ther. 2009;13(1):1–9.
11. Martin AM, Nolan D, Gaudieri S, et al. Predisposition to abacavir hypersensitivity conferred by HLA-B*5701 and a haplotypic Hsp70-Hom variant. Proc Natl Acad Sci. 2004;101(12):4180–4185.
12. Coleman JW. Protein haptenation by drugs. Clin Exp Allergy. 1998;28(Supp 4): 79–82.

13. LaRosa SP. Sepsis: Menu of new approaches replaces one therapy for all. *Cleve Clin J Med.* 2002;69:65–73.
14. Walensky RP, Goldberg JH, Daily JP. Anaphylaxis after rechallenge with abacavir. *AIDS.* 1999;28:999–1000.
15. Hewitt RG. Abacavir hypersensitivity reaction. *Clin Infect Dis.* 2002;34:1137–1142.
16. Martin MA, Klein TE, Dong BJ, Pirmohamed M, Haas DW, Kroetz DL. Clinical Pharmacogenetics Implementation Consortium guidelines for HLA-B genotype and abacavir dosing. *Clin Pharmacol Ther.* 2012;91(4):734–738.

Chapter **5**

Carbamazepine

LEARNING OBJECTIVES

Upon completion of this chapter, the student will be able to:

1. Recognize the genotype related to carbamazepine-induced Stevens-Johnson syndrome (SJS) and toxic epidermal necrolysis (TEN).
2. Explain the appropriate use of genetic testing in an individual who is to receive carbamazepine.
3. Interpret and utilize genetic-testing information relative to carbamazepine.

> The student should understand the potential for a gene–drug interaction related to adverse events seen in specific populations, even in the absence of individual genetic testing data for a given patient. The student also should understand that a valid genetic test can indicate a patient's risk of experiencing a severe adverse event, with the actionable response being an alternative drug therapy.

CASE QUESTIONS

Upon completion of this chapter, the student will be able to answer the following questions pertaining to the case of WH:

1. Would genetic testing for the HLA-B*15:02 allele be warranted in WH?
2. Could oxcarbazepine be used instead of carbamazepine in the Asian population?

Key Terms	
pharmacodynamic	The relationship between drug exposure and pharmacologic response.

Introduction

WH is a 17-year-old African American/Asian male with a history of head trauma suffered four months earlier in a motor vehicle accident (MVA). Recently, he was removed from his study hall at high school and sent to the school administrators because of teacher and student complaints of unprovoked aggressiveness and agitation, which were viewed as behavioral problems. WH visited his family physician, who referred WH to a neurologist. WH's mother states that the aggression and agitation have been increasing in recent months. The neurologist makes the diagnosis of acquired brain injury following examination of a CT scan.

WH is an active young man who participates in extracurricular activities and was always considered to be "happy-go-lucky." He is an average student and has many friends whom he has met through school and other activities. He has an unremarkable medical history, except for a broken arm, broken collarbone, and closed head trauma sustained in the MVA. He does not take any medication, but he has used creatine and whey protein as "supplements" to his wrestling workouts. WH is of African and Asian descent. As WH was adopted, there is minimal family history information.

The diagnosis of acquired brain injury is discussed, and the neurologist decides to start WH on carbamazepine for the treatment of agitation and aggression caused by the closed head trauma.[1] In consultation with the pharmacist, genetic testing for the human leukocyte antigen (HLA)-B*15:02 allele is undertaken, because there is a strong association between carbamazepine use and Stevens-Johnson syndrome (SJS) and toxic epidermal necrolysis (TEN) in individuals expressing the HLA-B*15:02 allele.[2–4]

Carbamazepine Pharmacodynamics

The influence of genetics relative to carbamazepine is in reference to potentially severe/life-threatening skin disorders that can occur with exposure to the drug. Stevens-Johnson syndrome and TEN have been observed as **pharmacodynamic** responses in patients receiving carbamazepine.[2-5] Stevens-Johnson syndrome initially presents as a febrile illness with stomatitis, purulent conjunctivitis, and skin lesions.[6] The syndrome, a hypersensitivity reaction, can be mild, resulting in fever, general malaise, and itching, with multiple lesions of the skin. The lesions may have the appearance of hives and may be papular or macular in nature with blisters. These lesions may be found on the trunk and arms and hands, including the palms, and the legs and feet, typically occurring symmetrically.[7] The severe form of SJS is necrotic skin occurring on less than 10% of a patient's body surface area (BSA).[8] Extensive necrotic lesions covering more than 30% of a patient's BSA is considered TEN.[9] This medical emergency is marked by full-thickness epidermal necrosis and involves the mucous membranes, with mortality reaching 40%.[10]

The hypersensitivity reaction resulting from exposure to carbamazepine is related to HLA- B*15:02, which is part of the human major histocompatibility complex (MHC). The MHC protein molecules that are expressed on cell surfaces work to help the body distinguish between its own cells and "foreign" cells. Although the mechanism of carbamazepine-induced SJS and TEN has not been confirmed, it has been hypothesized that some patients metabolize the drug in such a way that it results in the formation of metabolites that alter cellular proteins.[11] It is suggested that the altered proteins are recognized as foreign, resulting in the cellular (T-cell mediated) immune response that leads to SJS and TEN.

Chapter Summary

It is clear that the Asian population is at higher risk than other populations in regards to the potential for TEN and SJS with the administration of carbamazepine. Genotyping of individuals of Asian ethnicity would be prudent when considering the risk/benefit ratio of the use of carbamazepine. With respect to genotyping of other populations, again, the risk/benefit is to be considered. Here, the risk of TEN and SJS may be lower, and the need for carbamazepine versus other therapy is considered in this context. In patients with HLA-B*15:02, oxcarbazepine does not appear to be a choice as an alternative to carbamazepine as skin reactions have been noted in this population.[13,14] Guidelines for the use of carbamazepine relative to HLA-B*15:02 expression are currently being developed by the Clinical Pharmacogenetics Implementation Consortium.[15]

Genetic–Dynamic Interface: Carbamazepine Toxicity

Carbamazepine toxicity, with respect to SJS and TEN, is related to HLA-B*15:02. The frequency of the HLA-B*15:02 allele is dependent on the population. Table 5-1 presents the frequencies observed in various populations.

Table 5-1

HLA-B*15:02 Allele Frequencies in Major North American Populations

Ethnicity	Allele Frequency (%)	n
Asian	5.1	396
African	0.2	251
European	0	287
Hispanic	0	240

Source: Adapted from Ferrell PB McLeod HL. Carbamazepine, HLA-B*1502, and risk of Stevens-Johnson syndrome and toxic epidermal necrolysis: U.S. FDA recommendations. *Pharmacogenomics.* 2008;9(10):1543–1546.

The high frequencies of HLA-B*15:02 in the Asian population (e.g., Chinese) warrant pharmacogenetic testing prior to use of carbamazepine. In fact, a Black Box Warning has been added to the package labeling for the drug.[12] It states:

> Serious and sometimes fatal dermatologic reactions, including toxic epidermal necrolysis (TEN) and Sevens-Johnson syndrome (SJS), have been reported during treatment with carbamazepine. These reactions are estimated to occur in 1 to 6 per 10,000 new users in countries with mainly Caucasian populations, but the risk in some Asian countries is estimated to be about 10 times higher. Studies in patients of Chinese ancestry have found a strong association between the risk of developing SJS/TEN and the presence of HLA-B*1502, an inherited allelic variant of the HLA-B gene. HLA-B*1502 is found almost exclusively in patients with ancestry across broad areas of Asia.
>
> Patients with ancestry in genetically at-risk populations should be screened for the presence of HLA-B*1502 prior to initiating treatment with carbamazepine. Patients testing positive for the allele should not be treated with carbamazepine unless the benefit clearly outweighs the risk.

Answers to Case Questions

1. An individual with the HLA-B*15:02 allele is at increased risk for developing SJS and TEN. Although approximately 1 to 6 new Caucasian patients per 10,000 placed on carbamazepine experience these detrimental adverse events, some Asian populations incur a 10-fold higher risk (i.e., 10 to 60 Asian patients per 10,000).[12] With WH's Asian background, testing for the HLA-B*15:02 allele is warranted.

2. A small study indicated that a low dose of oxcarbazepine administered to each of three carbamazepine-sensitive patients resulted in skin reactions.[13] Additionally, a pilot study of oxcarbazepine showed a possible relationship between the presence of the HLA-B*15:02 allele and a skin reaction, characterized as maculopapular eruption.[14] It stands that oxcarbazepine may not be a clear alternative for use in Asian patients.

Review Questions

1. Carbamazepine toxicity expressed as SJS and TEN has been related to which of the following?
   a. CYP2C19*1/*2
   b. HLA-C*14:29
   c. VKORC1 A/G
   d. HLA-B*15:02
   e. HLA-B*57:01

2. Which of the following populations are most at risk for SJS when being treated with carbamazepine?
   a. Han Chinese
   b. North American African
   c. North American Asian
   d. a and c
   e. All of the above

3. Oxcarbazepine can be used as a therapeutic equivalent to carbamazepine because data show that it does not cause a skin reaction in patients with the HLA-B*15:02 allele.
   a. True
   b. False

4. The relationship between carbamazepine and the genetic constitution of an individual with regard to HLA allele status is an example of a:
   a. genetic–pharmacokinetic relationship.
   b. genetic–pharmacodynamic relationship.
   c. genetic–pharmacogenomic relationship.
   d. genetic–metabolic relationship.

5. Patients of Asian descent should be screened for the HLA-B*15:02 allele prior to the use of carbamazepine.
   a. True
   b. False

References

1. Azouvi P, Jokic C, Attal N, Denys P, Markabi S, Bussel B. Carbamazepine in agitation and aggressive behaviour following severe closed-head injury: results of an open trial. Brain Inj. 1999;13(10):797–804.

2. Chen P, Lin JL, Lu CS, et al. Carbamazepine-induced toxic effects and HLA-B*1502 screening in Taiwan. N Engl J Med. 2011;364:1126–1133.

3. Man CBL, Kwan P, Baum L, et al. Association between HLA-B*1502 allele and antiepileptic drug-induced cutaneous reactions in Han Chinese. Epilepsia. 2007;48(5):1015–1018.

4. Locharernkul C, Loplumlert J, Limotai C, et al. Carbamazepine and phenytoin induced Stevens-Johnson syndrome is associated with HLA-B*1502 allele in Thai. *Epilepsia.* 2008;49(12):2087–2091.

5. Ferrell PB, McLeod HL. Carbamazepine, HLA-B*1502, and risk of Stevens-Johnson syndrome and toxic epidermal necrolysis: U.S. FDA recommendations. *Pharmacogenomics.* 2008;9(10):1543–1546.

6. Stevens AM, Johnson FC. A new eruptive fever associated with stomatitis and ophthalmia: Report of two cases in children. *Am J Dis Child.* 1922;24:526–533.

7. Smelik M. Stevens-Johnson syndrome: A case study. *Permenente J.* 2002;6(1). Available at: http://xnet.kp.org/permanentejournal/winter02/casestudy.html. Accessed November 7, 2011.

8. Treat J. Stevens-Johnson syndrome and toxic epidermal necrolysis. *Ped Annal.* 2010;39(10):667–674.

9. Bastuji-Garin S, Rzany B, Stern RS, Shear NH, Naldi L, Roujeau JC. Clinical classification of cases of toxic epidermal necrolysis, Stevens-Johnson syndrome, and erythema multiforme. *Arch Dermatol.* 1993;129(1):92–96.

10. Lee A, Thompson J. Drug-induced skin reactions. In: Lee A (ed.). *Adverse drug reactions.* 2nd ed. Philadelphia, PA: Pharmaceutical Press; 2005: 125–156.

11. The Merck Manual. Stevens-Johnson Syndrome (SJS) and Toxic Epidermal Necrolysis (TEN). Available at: www.merckmanuals.com/professional/dermatologic_disorders/hypersensitivity_and_inflammatory_disorders/stevens Johnson_syndrome_sjs_and_toxic_epidermal_ necrolysis_ten.html. Accessed December 20, 2011.

12. Tegretol (carbamazepine) prescribing information. Available at: www.accessdata.fda.gov/drugsatfda_docs/label/2009/016608s101,018281s048lbl.pdf. Accessed November 4, 2011.

13. Beran RG. Cross-reactive skin eruption with both carbamazepine and oxcarbazepine. *Epilepsia.* 1993;34:163–165.

14. Hu FY, Wu XT, An DM, Yan B, Zhou D. Pilot association study of oxcarbazepine-induced mild cutaneous adverse reactions with HLA-B*1502 allele in Chinese Han population. *Seizure.* 2011;20(2):160–162.

15. PharmGKB. Gene–drug pairs. Available at: http://www.pharmgkb.org/page/cpicGeneDrugPairs. Accessed July 29, 2012.

Chapter **6**

Clopidogrel

LEARNING OBJECTIVES

Upon completion of this chapter, the student will be able to:

1. Recognize the various genotypes of cytochrome P450-2C19 (CYP2C19), relative to the prodrug clopidogrel.
2. Explain the appropriate use of genetic testing in an individual who is to receive clopidogrel.
3. Interpret and utilize genetic testing information relative to clopidogrel.

> Students should understand the potential for gene–drug interactions with regard to drug metabolizing enzymes, recognizing that variation in a drug metabolizing enzyme can affect the formation of an active compound. The student will understand that a valid genetic test can be utilized in assessing a patient's risk of therapeutic failure and the potential for severe complications. The student should understand that a patient's genotype may result in the actionable response of selecting an alternative therapeutic agent.

CASE QUESTIONS

Upon completion of this chapter, the student will be able to answer the following questions pertaining to the case of JK:

1. Based on JK's genetic information, would a standard 75 mg dose of clopidogrel be sufficient?
2. How might the pharmacist explain to JK the need for genetic screening and what her results mean?

Key Terms	
area under the curve (AUC; amt/vol · time)	A measure of drug exposure as the integrated area under the plasma drug concentration versus time curve from time zero to infinity.
bioavailability (F)	The rate and extent of drug absorption; the fraction of the dose reaching systemic circulation unchanged.
CYP; CYP450	The cytochrome P450 oxidative metabolic enzyme superfamily.
efflux transporter	A protein that moves drug out of cells/tissues.
extensive metabolizer (EM)	In general, an individual with two "normal-function" alleles relative to a drug metabolizing enzyme.
genotype	The specific set of alleles inherited at a locus on a given gene.
intermediate metabolizer (IM)	In general, an individual with one "loss-of-function" or one "reduced-function" allele and one "normal-function" allele relative to a drug metabolizing enzyme.
loading dose (D_L; amt)	The initial dose of a drug; administered with the intent of producing a near steady-state average concentration.
phenotype	An individual's expression of a physical trait or physiologic function due to genetic makeup and environmental and other factors.
poor metabolizer (PM)	An individual with two "reduced-function" or "loss-of-function" alleles relative to a drug metabolizing enzyme.
prodrug	A drug that requires conversion to an active form.
ultrarapid metabolizer (UM)	An individual with a "gain-of-function" allele, resulting in overexpression of a drug metabolizing enzyme.

Key Equations	
$$C_{ave}^{ss} = \frac{F \cdot Dose}{CL \cdot \tau}$$	The average steady-state drug concentration being directly related to the bioavailability and the dose and inversely related to the clearance and the dosing inverval.
$\uparrow, \downarrow$	The number of arrows indicates the relative difference in the magnitude of the change.

Introduction

JK is a 55-year-old white female who has just undergone percutaneous coronary intervention with coronary artery stent placement. JK has a five year history of type 2 diabetes that is well controlled. She also has a 10-year history of hypertension. JK's family history includes her father's passing at age 84 from a myocardial infarction and her mother's history of hyperlipidemia and hypertension. JK is placed on dual-antiplatelet therapy, including aspirin and clopidogrel. She agrees to have her genetic information screened for potential variants that could affect her clopidogrel therapy. Her genetic screening reveals a single nucleotide polymorphism (SNP) of cytochrome P450-2C19 (**CYP**2C19), indicating that she is homozygous for the *2 "loss-of-function" allele (*2/*2). This means that JK is a **poor metabolizer (PM)**. Thus, clopidogrel therapy may not work for JK, because CYP2C19 is responsible for the bioactivation of clopidogrel, which is a **prodrug**. Her physician wants to start her on a standard 75 mg/day dose of clopidogrel daily. Understanding that JK's genotype would negatively affect the use of clopidogrel, the pharmacist works with the physician to optimize JK's antiplatelet therapy.

Excessive coagulation and platelet aggregation are associated with the pathophysiology of numerous cardiovascular disorders, including myocardial infarctions, stroke, and occlusions of stents placed in coronary arteries as percutaneous coronary intervention(s). When the endothelial lining is damaged or a rough surface is exposed, circulating von Willebrand factor (vWF) binds to the exposed collagen. Clotting factor VIII is transported via the much larger protein vWF, with the two circulating as a complex. Factor VIII is synthesized in the liver, whereas vWF is synthesized in the endothelial cells. Factor VIII takes part in the coagulation cascade by activating factor X. Von Willebrand factor induces adhesion of platelets to subendothelial collagen via the glycoprotein (GpIb) platelet receptor. Platelet aggregation results from the formation of a fibrin bridge between the platelets at the GpIIb/IIIa receptor complex. Platelet adhesion is the binding of platelets to damaged endothelium or rough surfaces, while platelet aggregation is the binding of platelets to platelets (see **Figure 6-1**). Clopidogrel is an inhibitor of platelet aggregation.

Clopidogrel Pharmacodynamics

Clopidogrel is an inhibitor of platelet aggregation that works by irreversibly binding to the platelet adenosine diphosphate (ADP) $P2Y_{12}$ receptor. As stated previously, clopidogrel is a prodrug that requires bioactivation to elicit its therapeutic benefits.[1,2] In vitro, clopidogrel

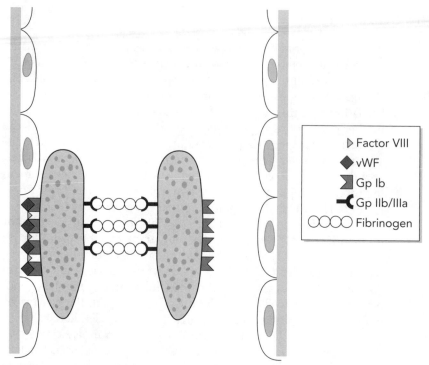

Figure 6-1 Adhesion (a) of platelets to subendothelial collagen via the glycoprotein (Gp Ib) platelet receptor. Platelet aggregation (b) occurs as a result of a fibrin bridge forming between the platelets at the Gp IIb/IIIa receptor complex. Clopidogrel inhibits platelet aggregation.

itself is not active as a platelet inhibitor. Cytochrome P450-2C19 is responsible for the biotransformation that yields a short-lived active metabolite that binds to the $P2Y_{12}$ receptor (see **Figure 6-2** and **Figure 6-3**).[3] Recent studies have shown that SNPs resulting in the generation of "loss-of–function" CYP2C19 enzymes alter the pharmacologic actions of clopidogrel and result in a decrease in efficacy.[4–6] Such a decrease in efficacy can result in life-threatening therapeutic failures. Studies have shown that the genotyping of CYP2C19 identifies greater than 90% of poor metabolizers.[1] Up to 30% of patients demonstrate some level of resistance to clopidogrel.[7,8] Thus, identifying these SNPs prior to treatment can assist prescribers in determining the best pharmacologic treatment plan for each individual patient.

Receptors are potential sites for SNPs that may result in altered therapeutic outcomes. Single nucleotide polymorphisms and other polymorphisms in the $P2Y_{12}$ receptor have been investigated for their potential role in clopidogrel resistance. Although mutations in the $P2Y_{12}$ gene have been associated with congenital bleeding disorders, they have not been associated with clopidogrel resistance.[9,10]

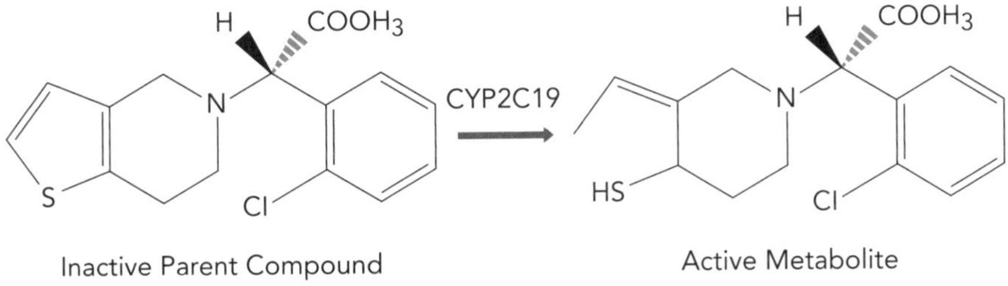

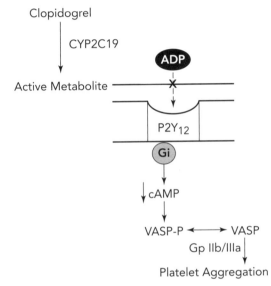

Figure 6-2 Clopidogrel is a thienopyridine molecule. CYP2C19 opens the thienopyridine ring structure exposing a sulfhydryl group for binding to the P2Y$_{12}$ receptor.

Figure 6-3 Clopidogrel is bioactivated by CYP2C19 to its active metabolite, which inhibits ADP binding to the P2Y$_{12}$ receptors on the platelet. When activated by ADP, the P2Y$_{12}$ removes a phosphate (P) from vasodilator stimulated phosphoprotein (VASP-P). VASP subsequently stimulates Gp IIb/IIIa receptor mediated platelet aggregation. The active metabolite of clopidogrel prevents ADP activation of the P2Y$_{12}$ receptor, which decreases platelet aggregation. However, if CYP2C19 contains a SNP decreasing clopidogrel bioactivation, platelet aggregation still occurs. Gi = inhibitory g-protein.

Clopidogrel Pharmacokinetics

The recommended oral maintenance dose of clopidogrel is 75 mg/day. At this dose, the peak therapeutic inhibition of platelet aggregation can be seen 3 to 7 days following drug initiation. **Loading doses** of 300 to 600 mg produce platelet inhibition within 3 to 5 hours. The peak plasma concentration of the parent and active metabolite occur in approximately one hour. Both the parent drug and the active metabolite are bound to protein in excess of 94%.[11] The intestinal absorption of clopidogrel is influenced by the **efflux transporter** P-glycoprotein (P-gp).[12] P-glycoprotein pumps drugs and other substances out of cells and, in the case of the gastrointestinal tract, back into the intestine for elimination in the feces. P-glycoprotein expression is encoded by the multidrug resistance gene MDR1. After a single loading dose of 300 or 600 mg of clopidogrel, patients who were homozygous for the MDR1 3435T variant were found to have lower C_{max} and **area under the curve (AUC)** values compared to controls. Food has been shown to increase the AUC of clopidogrel almost nine fold, and the terminal half-life doubles from 2.5 hours (fasting) to 5 hours (fed).[13] The half-life of the inactive metabolite is 8 hours. Clopidogrel is similarly eliminated in the feces (46%) and urine (50%).[14] Cytochrome P450-2C19 is responsible for the conversion of the parent drug to the active form. **Table 6-1** presents the CYP2C19 genotypes relative to drug metabolizing status.

Table 6-1

Cytochrome P450-2C19 Genotypes and Drug Metabolizing Status

Genotype	Metabolizing Status
*1/*1	Extensive metabolizer
*1/*17	Extensive metabolizer[a]
*17/*17	Ultrarapid metabolizer[a]
1/(2, 3, 4, 5, 6, 7, 8)	Intermediate metabolizer
(2[b], 3, 4, 5, 6, 7, 8)/(2, 3, 4, 5, 6, 7, 8)	Poor metabolizer

[a] Likely metabolizing status.

[b] Most common variant allele (G>681>A; 681G>A; rs4244285).

Genetic–Kinetic Interface: Clopidogrel

The prodrug clopidogrel is indicated for use in patients with acute coronary syndrome as an antiplatelet agent. The following is the Black Box Warning found in the trade name product (Plavix®) package labeling:[15]

Warning: Diminished Effectiveness in Poor Metabolizers

The effectiveness of Plavix is dependent on its activation to an active metabolite by the cytochrome P450 (CYP) system, principally CYP2C19. Plavix at recommended doses forms less of that metabolite and has a smaller effect on platelet function in patients who are CYP2C19 poor metabolizers. Poor metabolizers with acute coronary syndrome or undergoing percutaneous coronary intervention treated with Plavix at recommended doses exhibit higher cardiovascular event rates than do patients with normal CYP2C19 function. Tests are available to identify a patient's CYP2C19 genotype; these tests can be used as an aid in determining therapeutic strategy. Consider alternative treatment or treatment strategies in patients identified as CYP2C19 poor metabolizers.

A patient who is heterozygous, having the CYP2C19*1/*2 genotype, has intermediate metabolism of clopidogrel (one "normal-function" allele and one "loss-of-function" allele). It is expected that less of the active metabolite will be formed with a given standard dose and that more of the parent drug (clopidogrel) will reach systemic circulation, resulting in an increased concentration of the parent drug:

$$\uparrow C_{parent} = \frac{F \cdot Dose}{\downarrow CL}$$

Although the parent drug concentration will be increased, the efficacy of the drug will be decreased, because the active metabolite concentration (C_{active}) will be decreased. In this case, in a sense, as the **bioavailability (F)** of the active metabolite is decreased, the concentration of the active compound is decreased:

$$\downarrow C_{active} = \frac{\downarrow F \cdot Dose}{CL}$$

Clopidogrel Dosing

In 2010, the FDA issued a Black Box Warning on the prescribing information for clopidogrel.[15] This warning addresses the reduced effectiveness in patients who are poor metabolizers of clopidogrel and informs healthcare professionals that genetic tests are available for identification of genetic differences in CYP2C19. Cytochrome P450-2C19 has a number of "loss-of-function" alleles (*2, *3, *4, *5, *6, *7, and *8) and one gain-of-function allele (*17). The *2 "loss-of-function" allele is the most common, being present in greater than 90% of individuals with a variant form of the enzyme.

Patients who are **extensive metabolizers** (EM; *1/*1) have demonstrated an enhanced inhibition of platelet aggregation as compared to **intermediate metabolizers** [*1/*(2, 3, 4, 5, 6, 7, 8)]. Platelet inhibition is greater in intermediate metabolizers than in poor metabolizers (combination of two "loss-of-function" alleles, e.g. *2/*3).[16] Therefore, although standard doses would be sufficient in extensive metabolizers, intermediate metabolizers would necessarily require a higher dose of clopidogrel and alternative therapy should be considered. In poor metabolizers, those who are homozygous for two "loss-of-function" alleles, alternative platelet aggregation inhibitors should be utilized.

Drugs that are known inhibitors of CYP2C19 (e.g., the proton pump inhibitor lansoprazole) should be avoided in patients requiring therapeutic antiplatelet effects. Inhibitors of metabolism effectively make the patient a poor metabolizer. Clinicians need to recognize the potential for gene–drug interactions and also understand the influence of a drug–drug interaction in patients with a certain genotype (i.e., gene–drug–drug interaction). A thorough evaluation of the potential for significant interaction must accommodate the influence of more than one drug in the context of the individual's genetic characteristics. An example of a gene–drug–drug interaction is shown in **Figure 6-4**. Here, the extent of conversion of clopidogrel to its active form is dependent on the patient's genotype, with patients having a *1/*1 genotype being normal extensive metabolizers. With the addition of lansoprazole, a CYP2C19 inhibitor, the concentrations of the active metabolite of clopidogrel will decrease, and a higher than normal dose of clopidogrel will be required to obtain therapeutic benefit. However, if lansoprazole is added to therapy in an intermediate metabolizer, the additional inhibition of clopidogrel bioactivation would result in little to no active drug being formed and would likely result in therapeutic failure. In this case, the patient would have the phenotype of a poor metabolizer but the genotype of an intermediate metabolizer.

An individual's CYP2C19 genotype can indicate the therapeutic response to clopidogrel. With more than 29 million prescriptions for clopidogrel written in 2010 and more than 28 million in 2011, and with genotyping not being included in the current standard of care, it is likely that some patients (i.e., intermediate and poor metabolizers) are not receiving the full therapeutic benefit from the drug, and some may not be receiving any benefit.[17] The Clinical Pharmacogenetics

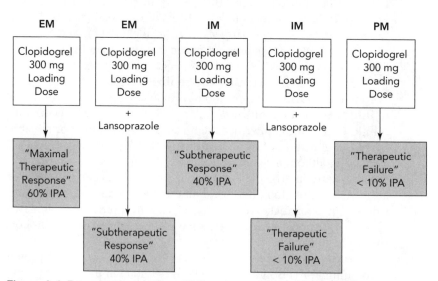

Figure 6-4 Extensive metabolizer (EM) patients administered a 300 mg dose of clopidogrel will obtain a maximal therapeutic response of 60% inhibition of platelet aggregation (IPA). The addition of lansoprazole pharmacologically inhibits CYP2C19, making the EM patient appear like an IM patient. The addition of lansoprazole to an IM patient results in therapeutic failure in a fashion similar to a PM patient.

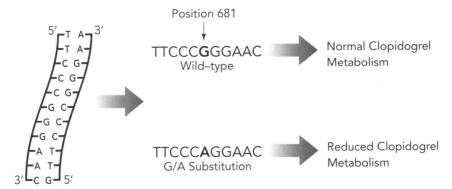

Figure 6-5 Example SNP related to CYP2C19*2 resulting in reduced clopidogrel conversion (reduced metabolism of the prodrug) to the active form with potentially decreased therapeutic efficacy.
Note: On the continuous DNA strands, the first two bases are the last two of a codon, with subsequent codons following.

Implementation Consortium has published dosing guidelines related to the CYP2C19–clopidogrel gene–drug pair.[18] Additionally, the indication specific use of genotyping CYP2C19 in patients undergoing coronary artery stent placement has been clearly presented and explained relative to clopidogrel use.[19]

Chapter Summary

Genotyping of CYP2C19 in the face of clopidogrel therapy in patients with coronary artery stent placement may avoid the administration of the drug to patients who will not benefit from it. Identification of CYP2C19 intermediate and poor metabolizers will allow for the use of antiplatelet therapies with the potential for greater efficacy in patients having undergone stent placement. **Figure 6-5** presents an example of the genetic influence on clopidogrel metabolism relative to CYP2C19.

Answers to Case Questions

1. Because clopidogrel is a prodrug requiring bioactivation by CYP2C19, a standard 75 mg dose would not be sufficient. Because JK is homozygotic for the SNP in CYP2C19, she would not respond to clopidogrel even if the dose were doubled. She should be placed on an alternative antiplatelet agent.
2. When first discussing the need for genetic testing, JK needs to be reassured that she is only being screened to determine her likelihood of responding to clopidogrel, not her susceptibility to disease or anything else. The discussion should include

how genetic screening can help to save her life, determine the need for a therapeutic alternative, and save her money. Her genetic screening results should be explained to her such that she understands clopidogrel will not work for her and that alternative therapies are available.

Review Questions

1. If a patient has been identified with a SNP in CYP2C19 that results in decreased enzyme activity and has also been taking ketoconazole (an inhibitor of CYP2C19) for a fungal infection, what would you suggest for this patient if he or she was just given a prescription for a standard dose (75 mg once daily) of clopidogrel?
   a. Increase the starting dose.
   b. Decrease the starting dose.
   c. Maintain the normal starting dose.
   d. Switch to a drug other than clopidogrel.

2. A SNP in CYP2C19 may result in the decreased bioactivation of which of the following agents?
   a. Warfarin
   b. Clopidogrel
   c. Codeine
   d. Azathioprine
   e. None of the above

3. Platelet aggregation results from a fibrin bridge forming between platelets and the:
   a. $P2Y_{12}$ receptor.
   b. GpIIb/IIIa receptor.
   c. ADP receptor.
   d. GpIb receptor.

4. Which of the following is true of the FDA Black Box Warning on clopidogrel found in the package labeling?
   a. It warns that toxic concentrations of the active metabolite may accumulate in poor metabolizers.
   b. It informs healthcare professionals that tests are available to identify genetic differences in CYP2C19 function.
   c. It recommends doubling the dose of clopidogrel in poor metabolizers.
   d. All of the above.

5. Based on the following bar graph, which group of metabolizers has the highest exposure to active metabolite and the greatest platelet inhibition? (MPA = mean platelet aggregation)

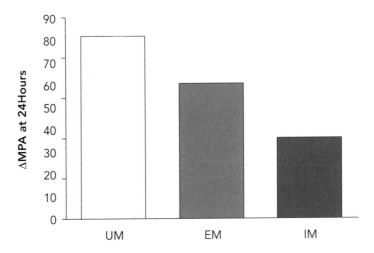

Clopidogrel, 600mg

a. Ultrarapid metabolizers
b. Extensive metabolizers
c. Intermediate metabolizers
d. All are exposed to the same concentration of active metabolite and have equal platelet inhibition.

References

1. Frere C, Cuisset T, Morange PE, et al. Effect of cytochrome p450 polymorphisms on platelet reactivity after treatment with clopidogrel in acute coronary syndrome. *Am J Cardiol.* 2008;101(8):1088–1093.
2. Storey RF. Clopidogrel in acute coronary syndrome: To genotype or not? *Lancet.* 2009;373(9660):276–278.
3. Gurbel PA, Tantry US. Clopidogrel resistance? *Throm Res.* 2007;120:311–321.
4. Mega JL, Close SL, Wiviott SD, et al. Cytochrome P-450 polymorphisms and response to clopidogrel. *N Eng J Med.* 2009;60(4):354–362.
5. Simon T, Verstuyft C, Mary-Krause M, et al. Genetic determinants of response to clopidogrel and cardiovascular events. *N Eng J Med.* 2009;360(4):363–375.
6. Collet JP, Hulot JS, Pena A, et al. Cytochrome P450 2C19 polymorphism in young patients treated with clopidogrel after myocardial infarction: A cohort study. *Lancet.* 2009;373(9660):309–337.
7. Nguyen TA, Diodati JG, Pharand C. Resistance to clopidogrel: A review of the evidence. *J Am Coll Cardiol.* 2003;91:1123–1125.

8. Wang TH, Bhatt DL, Topol EJ. Aspirin and clopidogrel resistance: An emerging clinical entity. Eur Heart J. 2006;27:647–654.
9. Conley PB, Delaney SM. Scientific and therapeutic insights into the role of the platelet P2Y12 receptor in thrombosis. Curr Opin Hematol. 2003;10:333–338.
10. Bonello L, Palot-Bonello N, Armero S, et al. Impact of loading dose adjustment on platelet reactivity in homozygotes of the 2C19*2 loss of function polymorphism. Int J. Cardiol. 2010;145(1):165–166.
11. Mullangi R, Srinivas NR. Clopidogrel: Review of bioanalytical methods, pharmacokinetics/pharmacodynamics, and update on recent trends in drug–drug interaction studies. Biomed Chromatogr. 2009;23:26–41.
12. Taubert D, vonBeckerath N, Grimberg G, et al. Impact of P-glycoprotein on clopidogrel absorption. Clin Pharmacol Ther. 2006;80:486–501.
13. Nirogi RV, Kandikere VN, Mudigonda K. Effect of food on bioavailability of a single dose of clopidogrel in healthy male subjects. Arzneimittelforschung. 2006;56:735–739.
14. Lins R, Broekhuysen J, Necciari J, Deroubaix X. Pharmacokinetic profile of 14C-labeled clopidogrel. Sem Thrombosis Hemostasis. 1999;25:29–33.
15. Plavix (clopidogrel) prescribing information. Available at: http://products .sanofi.us/plavix/plavix.html. Accessed April 17, 2012.
16. Kim KA, Park PW, Hong SJ, Park J-Y. The effects of CYP2C19 polymorphism on the pharmacokinetics and pharmacodynamics of clopidogrel: A possible mechanism for clopidogrel resistance. Clin Pharmacol Ther. 2008;84(2):236–242.
17. Bartholow M. Top 200 drugs of 2010. Pharmacy Times. Available at: www. pharmacytimes.com/publications/issue/2012/July2012/Top-200-Drugs -of-2011. Accessed August 3, 2012.
18. Scott SA, Sangkuhl K, Gardner EE, et al. Clinical Pharmacogenetics Implementation Consortium guidelines for cytochrome P450-2C19 (CYP2C19) genotype and clopidogrel therapy. Clin Pharmacol Ther. 2011;90(2):328–332.
19. Johnson JA, Roden DM, Lesko LJ, Ashley E, Klein TE, Shuldiner AR. Clopidogrel: A case for indication-specific pharmacogenetics. Clin Pharmacol Ther. 2012;91(5):774–776.

Chapter 7

5-Fluorouracil

LEARNING OBJECTIVES

Upon completion of this chapter, the student will be able to:

1. Recognize the various genotypes of dihydropyrimidine dehydrogenase (DPD) relative to 5-fluorouracil metabolism.
2. Explain the appropriate use of genetic testing in an individual who is to receive 5-fluorouracil.
3. Interpret and apply genetic testing information relative to 5-fluorouracil.

> Students should understand the potential for a gene–drug interaction with regard to drug metabolizing enzymes, recognizing that variation in a metabolizing enzyme, if not understood, can lead to severe toxicity and death. Students should understand that a valid genetic test can indicate a patient's risk of toxicity, allowing for the actionable

response of dose adjustment or the use of a different therapeutic agent.

CASE QUESTIONS

Upon completion of this chapter, the student will be able to answer the following questions pertaining to the case of NC:

1. Based on NC's genetic constitution, would a standard dose of 5-fluorouracil be warranted?
2. How might the pharmacist explain to NC the need for genetic screening and what her results mean?

Key Terms	
area under the curve (AUC; amt/vol · time)	A measure of drug exposure as the integrated area under the plasma drug concentration versus time curve from time zero to infinity.
clearance (CL; vol/time)	The volume of biologic fluid from which drug is removed per unit time.
pharmacodynamic	The relationship between drug exposure and pharmacologic response.
prodrug	A drug that requires conversion to an active form.

Key Equations	
$t_{\frac{1}{2}} = \dfrac{0.693 \times Vd}{CL} = \dfrac{0.693}{k_e}$	The half-life, being directly related to the volume of distribution and inversely related to the clearance; inversely related to the elimination rate constant, k_e.
$AUC = \dfrac{Dose}{CL}$	The area under the concentration versus time curve, being proportional to the dose and inversely proportional to the clearance.
$\uparrow, \downarrow$	The number of arrows indicates the relative difference in the magnitude of the change.

Introduction

NC is an anxious 39-year-old Caucasian female who presents to the oncology clinic upon referral. While performing a monthly breast self-exam, NC found a lump in the lower outer quadrant of her right breast. NC subsequently saw her gynecologist, who also felt the hard, mobile mass in the described location. There was no associated skin change, pain, or discharge. Mammography was ordered, with the plan to biopsy any suspicious lesions. The mammogram identified a suspicious mass, a core biopsy was performed, and results were positive for malignancy. NC was referred to the oncology clinic for further evaluation and discussion of treatment options. NC began menses at age 11. She has a 7-year-old daughter and is currently taking birth control pills (started at age 18, stopped for pregnancy, and then resumed). Additionally, NC has a history of anxiety and frequent migraines (more than two per month). Her mother was diagnosed with breast cancer at age 54; she is currently 62. Her maternal aunt died of breast cancer at age 46, and her maternal grandmother died of the disease at age 54. NC denies pain or discomfort but complains of frequent urination and "feeling ill." A computed tomography (CT) scan of the abdomen and a bone scan were negative for metastases.

The core biopsy shows a histological grade of G1, estrogen receptor–positive tissue (90%) with FISH − 2+ HER2/neu overexpression. Additionally, sentinel lymph node biopsy identified the involvement of two axillary nodes, both of which exhibited movement. Pharmacogenetic testing indicates that NC is heterozygotic for an allele (DPD*2A) that results in inactive dihydropyrimidine dehydrogenase (DPD).

Purines and pyrimidines are the building blocks of deoxyribonucleic acid (DNA) and ribonucleic acid (RNA). During tumor growth and proliferation, DNA and RNA synthesis is accelerated, increasing the cell's demand for pyrimidines. 5-Fluorouracil (5-FU) is a pyrimidine analog that replaces pyrimidines during DNA and RNA replication.[1] Therapeutic agents that interfere with purine and pyrimidine synthesis and that are structurally similar to these endogenous compounds are classified as antimetabolites. Colon, breast, and upper gastrointestinal (GI) carcinomas respond to the antimetabolite 5-FU.

5-Fluorouracil Pharmacodynamics

Once transported into the tumor cell, 5-FU is converted through a series of enzymatic reactions to its active metabolite, 5-fluorodeoxyuridine monophosphate (FdUMP). This active metabolite forms a tight covalent complex with thymidylate synthase in the presence of the folate cofactor 5,10-methylene tetrahydrofolate. Thymidylate synthase catalyzes the methylation of dUMP to dTMP, an essential step in DNA synthesis (see **Figure 7-1**). Because 5-FU is incorporated into both DNA and RNA, RNA processing is also altered.

5-fluorouracil toxicity typically consists of anorexia, nausea, vomiting, and stomatitis. In patients with DPD deficiency, these toxicities are drastically increased, resulting in GI ulcerations, diarrhea, neutropenia, neuropathy, shock, and potentially death.

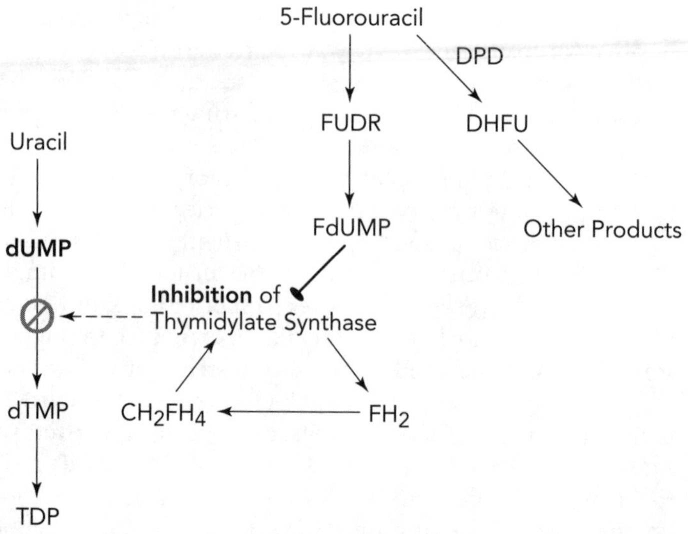

Figure 7-1 The proposed primary mechanism of action of 5-Fluorouracil. 5-FU (via FdUMP) inhibits thymidylate synthase, an enzyme required for the methylation of uracil to deoxyuridine monophosphate (dUMP) to deoxythymidine monophosphate (dTMP). TDP = thymidine diphosphate; FH_2 = dihydrofolate; CH_2FH_4 = methyl tetrahyrdofolate. 5-Fluorouracil is metabolized by dihydropyrimidine dehydrogenase (DPD) to form dihydrofluorouracil (DHFU). A SNP resulting in inactive DPD can result in 5-FU severe toxicity and death in the face of standard dosing.

5-Fluorouracil Pharmacokinetics

Dihydropyrimidine dehydrogenase is the rate-limiting enzyme in the catabolism of 5-FU (Figure 7-1; see **Figure 7-2**). Catabolism is a form of metabolism that results in the breakdown of a molecule and the release of energy. Dihydropyrimidine dehydrogenase has been found to be responsible for 80% of the catabolism of 5-FU, which mainly occurs in the liver. A single nucleotide polymorphism (SNP) in the DPD gene (DPYD) has been shown to result in a DPD enzyme without catabolic activity.[2] This SNP consists of a G → A mutation changing an invariant GT splice donor site into AT, which leads to skipping of a 165 base pair exon. Ultimately, this results in the amino acid residues 581-635 in the DPD protein being incorporated incorrectly into the enzyme, causing a lack of activity. This DPD*2A variant is the most common mutation observed in cancer patients and has been reported to be present in 1.8% of the Dutch population.[3,4] A reduction in DPD activity has been shown to increase the elimination half-life ($t_{1/2}$) and **area under the curve (AUC)** of 5-FU.[5,6] 5-FU is administered via the parenteral route. Following an IV dose, it has a plasma half-life of 10 to 20 minutes. Less than 10% of the drug is excreted unchanged

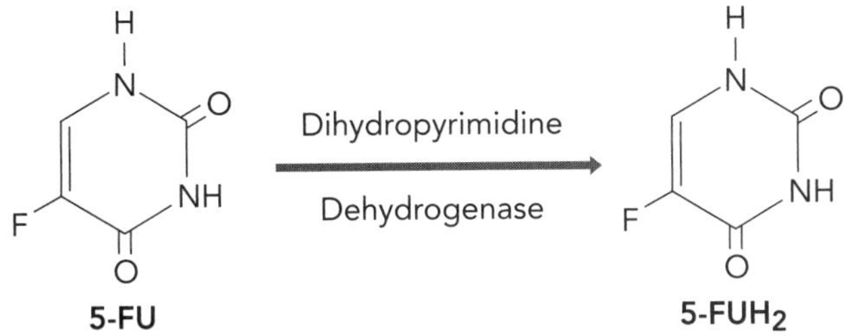

Figure 7-2 The initial and rate-limiting step in the catabolism of 5-FU is dihydropyrimidine dehydrogenase (DPD) mediated reduction of 5-FU to dihydrofluorouracil (DHFU, 5-FUH$_2$).

in the urine. Continuous IV infusion of 300–500 mg/m^2 per day results in peak concentrations of 11.2 μM.[7] The prolonged half-life and increased AUC in DPD deficiency results in increased exposure to 5-FU, which leads to adverse events.

In order to produce a synergistic **pharmacodynamic** response, 5-FU is typically given with other chemotherapeutic agents, such as irinotecan, cyclophosphamide, or methotrexate. A reduced form of folic acid, leucovorin, may also be coadministered to stabilize FdUMP binding to thymidylate synthase.

Genetic–Kinetic Interface: 5-FU Catabolism

5-FU is a **prodrug** that must be converted to the active antimetabolite. Through pyrimidine salvage pathways, 5-FU is catabolized to produce active metabolites. The rate-limiting step in the catabolism of 5-FU is the DPD-mediated conversion of 5-FU to dihydrofluorouracil (DHFU). A deficiency in DPD, as is seen with the DPD*2A variant, results in a decreased **clearance (CL)** of 5-FU, leading to increased exposure:

$$\uparrow AUC = \frac{\textit{5-FUDose}}{\downarrow CL}$$

The decreased clearance also results in a longer half-life of 5-FU:

$$\uparrow t_{\frac{1}{2}} = \frac{0.693 \cdot V}{\downarrow CL}$$

Thus, a standard dose of 5-FU in patients deficient in DPD results in increased exposure, which can result in increased risk of toxicity and death. Those heterozygous for DPD*2A have decreased DPD function, whereas those who are homozygous have a lack of function and are at the highest risk of 5-FU toxicity.

Chapter Summary

Individuals who have a loss-of-function variant of DPD may experience severe (high-grade) toxicity with "normal dose" 5-FU administration. Genetic testing can identify individuals who would require a lower dose of 5-FU in order to avoid severe toxicity. Specific 5-FU dosing guidelines are being developed by the Clinical Pharmacogenetics

Implementation Consortium.[8] The Dutch Pharmacogenetics Working Group Guidelines recommends that individuals with one variant DPD allele should receive a dose that is 50% of the normal dose or should receive alternative therapy. Individuals with two variant alleles should receive an alternative therapy to 5-FU.[9]

Answers to Case Questions

1. A standard dose of 5-FU would not be appropriate for NC. In fact, NC would be at risk of increased toxicity if a standard dose was started. A lower-than-normal dose would be required for NC, specifically 50% of the standard dose. Another option may be use of a different therapeutic agent.[10]

2. The pharmacist should explain to NC that this genetic screening was performed to determine if she was a candidate to receive 5-FU. The pharmacist would want to explain that chemotherapeutic agents are associated with side effects that may limit their use in some patients. By screening for the DPD genotype, the healthcare team can determine if NC is a good candidate to receive 5-FU and determine an appropriate dose should 5-FU be utilized.

Review Questions

1. Which of the following is 5-FU's pharmacodynamic target?
   a. Dihydroxypyrimidine dehydrogenase
   b. Topoisomerase I
   c. Dihydrofolate reductase
   d. Thymidylate synthase

2. Which of the following is the rate-limiting enzyme in the catabolism of 5-FU?
   a. Dihydroxypyrimidine dehydrogenase
   b. Topoisomerase I
   c. Dihydrofolate reductase
   d. CYP2C19

3. 5-FU replaces a _____ during DNA and RNA replication.
   a. purine
   b. pyrimidine
   c. piperazine
   d. piperidine

4. A deficiency of DPD activity results in a(n) _____ in clearance and a(n) _____ in half-life of 5-FU.
   a. increase; increase
   b. decrease; decrease
   c. decrease; increase
   d. increase; no change

5. Which of the following is *not* a side effect of 5-FU toxicity?
   a. Dyspepsia
   b. Anorexia
   c. Nausea, vomiting, diarrhea
   d. Stomatitis

References

1. Daily Med fluorouracil package label. Available at: http://dailymed.nlm.nih.gov/dailymed/lookup.cfm?setid=b90e0da7-f702-4f09-9488-74f2bb20e9ac. Accessed July 26, 2012.

2. Wei X, McLeod HL, McMurrough J, Gonzalez FJ, Fernandez-Salguero P. Molecular basis of the human dihydropyrimidine dehydrogenase deficiency and 5-fluorouracil toxicity. *J Clin Invest.* 1996;98:610–615.

3. van Kuilenburg ABP, Vreken P, Beex LVAM, et al. Heterozygosity for a point mutation in an invariant splice donor site of dihydropyrimidine dehydrogenase and severe 5-fluorouracil related toxicity. *Eur J Cancer.* 1997;33:2258–2264.

4. van Kuilenburg ABP, Baars JW, R. Meinsma R, van Gennip AH. Lethal 5-fluorouracil toxicity associated with a novel mutation in the dihydropyrimidine dehydrogenase gene. *Ann Onc.* 2003;14(2):341–342.

5. Diasio RB, Beavers TL, Carpenter JT. Familial deficiency of dihydropyrimide dehydrogenase: Biochemical basis of familial pyrimidemia and severe 5-fluorouracil induced toxicity. *J Clin Invest.* 1988;81:47–51.

6. Maring JG, van Kuilenburg ABP, Haasjes J, et al. Reduced 5-FU clearance in a patient with low DPD activity due to heterozygosity for a mutant allele of the DPYD gene. *Br J Cancer.* 2002;86:1028–1033.

7. Diasio RB, Harris BE. Clinical pharmacology of 5-fluorouracil. *Clin Pharmacokinet.* 1989;16:215–237.

8. PharmGKB. Gene–drug pairs. Available at: www.pharmgkb.org/page/cpicGeneDrugPairs. Accessed July 29, 2012.

9. PharmGKB. Dutch Pharmacogenetics Working Group Guideline: Fluorouracil, DPYD. Available at: www.pharmgkb.org/gene/PA145. Accessed October 19, 2012.

10. Swen JJ, Nijenhuis M, de Boer A, et al. Pharmacogenetics: From bench to byte—an update of guidelines. *Clin Pharmacol Ther.* 2011;89(5):662–673.

Chapter **8**

Irinotecan

LEARNING OBJECTIVES

Upon completion of this chapter, the student will be able to:

1. Recognize the various genotypes of uridine diphosphate glucuronosyl-transferase (UGT1A) relative to irinotecan metabolism.
2. Describe the appropriate use of genetic testing in an individual who is to receive irinotecan.
3. Interpret and utilize genetic testing information relative to irinotecan.

> The student should understand that genetic variation can lead to altered conversion of a potentially toxic metabolite to an inactive form. Applying valid pharmacogenetic testing can aid in decision making relative to the actionable response of appropriate dosage adjustment in a given patient.

CASE QUESTIONS

Upon completion of this chapter, the student will be able to answer the following questions pertaining to the case of DT:

1. Based on DT's genetic constitution, would a standard dose of irinotecan be warranted?
2. How might the pharmacist explain to DT the need for genetic screening and what the results mean?

Key Terms	
clearance (CL; vol/time)	The volume of biologic fluid from which drug is removed per unit time.
genotype	The specific set of alleles inherited at a locus on a given gene.
pharmacogenetics (PGt)	The study of a gene involved in response to a drug.

Key Equations	
↑, ↓	The number of arrows indicates the relative difference in the magnitude of the change.

Introduction

DT is a 61-year-old African American male who presented to his primary care physician with complaints of abdominal discomfort and blood in his stool for the past four months. Upon physical examination, the physician noted a positive stool guaiac test and decreased hematocrit and hemoglobin compared with values obtained approximately 13 months ago during an annual physical examination. DT was referred to a gastroenterologist, and a subsequent colonoscopy revealed multiple polyps as well as a mass in his transverse colon. A staging computed tomography (CT) scan revealed metastatic disease to the liver. DT was diagnosed with Dukes' stage D colon cancer (stage IV disease), and the decision was made to surgically resect the transverse colon and regional lymph nodes. The surgeon also performed a colostomy. DT now presents to the oncology outpatient clinic for his first course of chemotherapy.

DT is a jeweler, specializing in Swiss watch repair. He has smoked a pipe for 30 years. He states that he drinks beer (12 to 24 oz. three times a week). DT is married with two adult children, all alive and well. He is planning to retire and move to Florida in two years. He currently takes the following medications: glyburide 5 mg by mouth twice daily (5 years); Gaviscon® one tablet by mouth before bedtime, as needed; and ranitidine 150 mg by mouth at bedtime (6 years).

DT agrees to have his genetic information screened for potential variants that could affect his current medication therapy. His genetic screening reveals a single nucleotide polymorphism (SNP) of uridine diphosphate glucuronosyltransferase (UGT1A1*28; homozygotic), which results in decreased enzyme expression.[1] His physician wants to start him on a standard dose of irinotecan. The pharmacist agrees to review **pharmacogenetics (PGt)** and medications with DT.

Cancer is a disease in which the cellular control mechanisms that govern proliferation and differentiation are changed. Drugs used in cancer chemotherapy target important biosynthetic processes in proliferating cells. The cell cycle (see **Figure 8-1**) demonstrates the phases of DNA replication and mitosis. During the G1 phase, the cell prepares for mitosis and begins DNA synthesis; it is a period of rapid growth and metabolic activity. Cells that are at rest but not prepar-

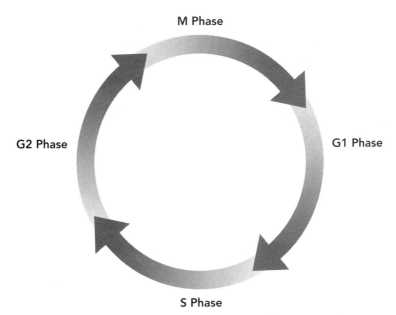

Figure 8-1 The cell cycle. The G1 phase represents cells preparing for mitosis and the beginning of DNA synthesis; it is a period of rapid growth and metabolic activity. Cells that are at rest but not preparing for cell division are in the G0 phase. (not shown). The S phase is the period of DNA synthesis and the target phase of many antitumor drugs, including irinotecan. G2 is a growth phase where the cell prepares for division. The M phase is the cellular division phase.

ing for cell division are in the G0 phase. The S phase is the period of DNA synthesis, and it is the target phase of many antitumor drugs, including irinotecan. G2 is the growth phase where the cell prepares for division. During the M phase, the cell divides.

Irinotecan Pharmacodynamics

During the S phase, the DNA double helix unwinds (see **Figure 8-2**). The unwinding of the DNA double helix results in torsional strain on the DNA strand, which is comparable to taking a tightly twisted rubber band and pulling it straight. If small cuts are made in the rubber band, the torsional strain is reduced. The cellular enzyme topoisomerase I (Top I) relieves this torsional strain in the DNA by creating reversible single-strand breaks. Irinotecan, which is indicated for the treatment of colorectal cancer, binds to Top I and prevents the repair of the single-strand breaks, thus stopping the S phase of the cell cycle.

Irinotecan and its hydrolyzation metabolite, SN-38, are active inhibitors of Top I.[2] SN-38 is more potent than irinotecan itself; as such, irinotecan is considered to be a prodrug.[3] Hydrolyzation of irinotecan to SN-38 occurs in the intestinal mucosa, the plasma, and primarily in the liver by carboxylesterase (see **Figure 8-3**). SN-38 is converted to an inactive metabolite by UGT1A.

The SN-38 active metabolite has been associated with dose-limiting toxicities, including myelosuppression and severe diarrhea.[4,5] Patients who are homozygous for the UGT1A1*28 allele are more susceptible to these dose-limiting toxicities due to a decreased conversion of SN-38 to an inactive metabolite. For this reason, a reduction in the starting dose of irinotecan should be considered for such patients.

Irinotecan Pharmacokinetics

Irinotecan is metabolized primarily by hepatic carboxylesterase to SN-38 (see Figure 8-3). The SN-38 active metabolite undergoes conjugation by uridine diphosphate (UDP-(UGT1A1)) to form an inactive glucuronide metabolite. Although smoking increases the formation of SN-38, it has a greater effect on SN-38 glucuronidation, resulting in overall lower levels of the SN-38 active metabolite.[6,7] SN-38 levels are increased by the UGT1A1*28 polymorphism due to decreased inactivation. Ten percent of North Americans are homozygous for the UGT1A1*28 allele. Seven TA repeats in the TATA box of the UGT1A1 promoter region results in the variant allele UGT1A1*28. Irinotecan

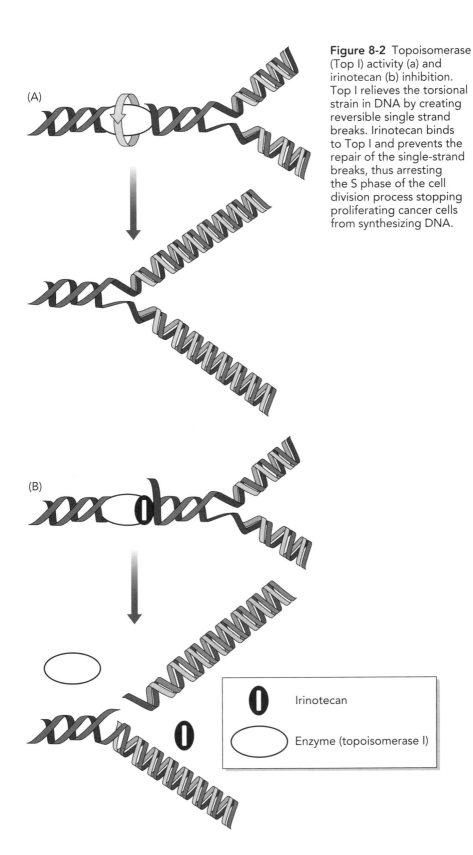

Figure 8-2 Topoisomerase (Top I) activity (a) and irinotecan (b) inhibition. Top I relieves the torsional strain in DNA by creating reversible single strand breaks. Irinotecan binds to Top I and prevents the repair of the single-strand breaks, thus arresting the S phase of the cell division process stopping proliferating cancer cells from synthesizing DNA.

(A)

(B)

0 Irinotecan

Enzyme (topoisomerase I)

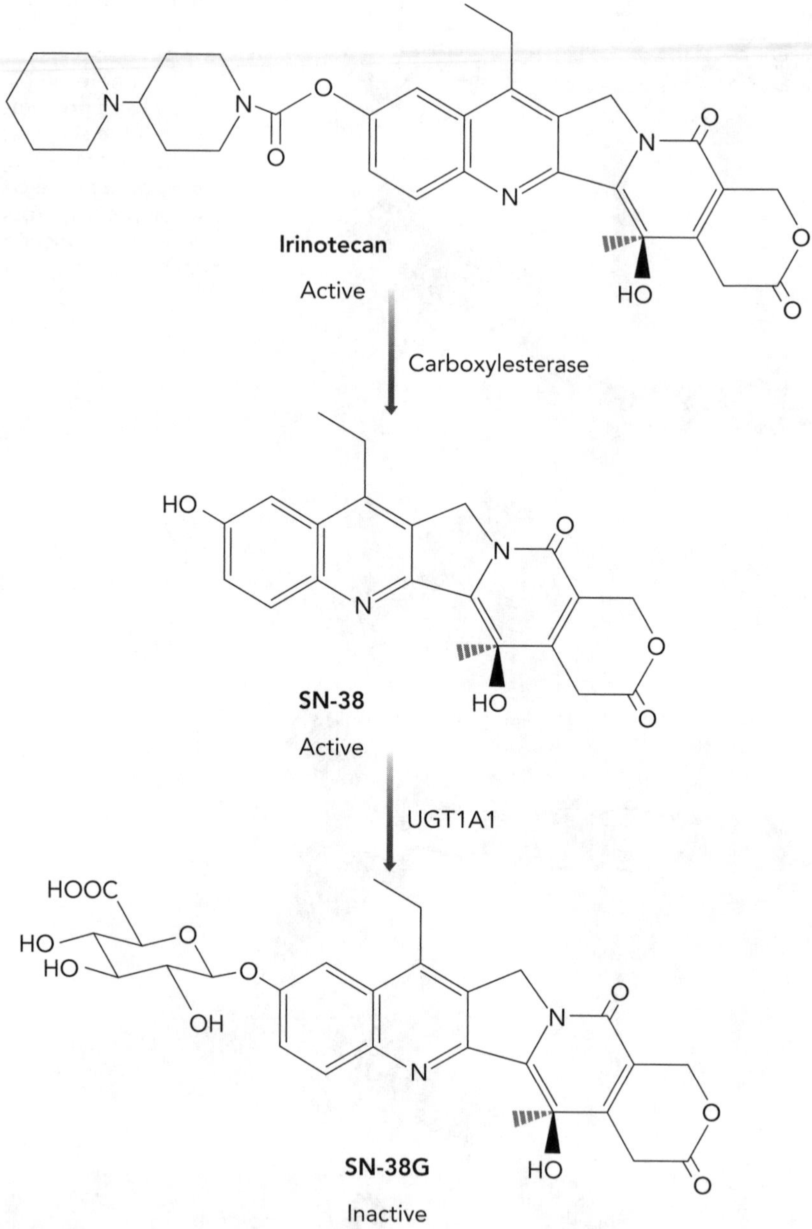

Figure 8-3 Irinotecan bioactivation to SN-38. Both the parent (irinotecan) and carboxylesterase metabolite (SN-38) are active Top I inhibitors; however, SN-38 is more active than irinotecan. The uridine diphosphate glucuronosyltransferase (UGT1A1) metabolite (SN-38G) is inactive.

has an elimination half-life of 6 to 12 hours, and the estimated half-life of SN-38 is 10 to 20 hours.

Genetic–Kinetic Interface: SN-38 Glucuronidation

Irinotecan is a prodrug that provides therapeutic concentrations of the active compound SN-38 in the blood. SN-38 can be eliminated from the body by glucuronidation via UGT1A1. An individual may have the genetic constitution that results in a decrease in the formation of SN-38 glucuronide and higher concentrations of SN-38, such as those with the UGT1A1*28 homology (*28/*28). In such cases, SN-38 concentrations are higher because the **clearance (CL)** of SN-38 via glucuronidation is decreased:

$$\uparrow C_{SN\text{-}38} = \frac{SN\text{-}38\,Dose}{CL \downarrow}$$

An individual who does not have the *28/*28 genetic constitution and who smokes may be expected to have an increased rate of formation of SN-38 from irinotecan, effectively increasing the "dose" of SN-38. Such individuals may also expect an increase in the glucuronidation of SN-38. It has been shown that smoking has a greater effect on the glucuronidation ($\uparrow\uparrow$) of SN-38 than it does on the formation ($\uparrow$) of SN-38:

$$\downarrow C_{SN\text{-}38} = \frac{\uparrow SN\text{-}38\,Dose}{CL \uparrow\uparrow}$$

Notably, it has been shown that smokers have a decreased risk of irinotecan-induced neutropenia as compared to nonsmokers.

The relationship between genetics and kinetics must always be taken into account. For instance, what would be expected to happen to the SN-38 concentration and side-effect profile of irinotecan in a *28/*28 individual who smokes?

A decrease in the starting dose of irinotecan is recommended for patients who have been found to be homozygous for the UGT1A1*28 allele. Clinical research on patients who are heterozygous for UGT1A1*28 has been variable for increased neutropenic risk, and such patients have tolerated normal starting doses. An FDA-approved test (Invader® UGT1A1 Molecular Assay) is available for clinical determination of the UGT **genotype**. Irinotecan is only commercially available for intravenous administration, with a weekly regimen of 125 mg/m^2 over 90 minutes on days 1, 8, 15, and 22 of a 6-week treatment cycle (may adjust upward to 150 mg/m^2, if tolerated). Other dosing regimens are also available for dosing in 3-week intervals or in combination with other chemotherapeutic agents. Additionally, a patient's history of cigarette smoking should be taken into consideration when initiating therapy with irinotecan. The Royal Dutch Pharmacists Association–Pharmacogenetics Working Group has offered dosing recommendations for irinotecan based on UGT1A1 genotype and the Clinical Pharmacogenetics Implementation Consortium plans to evaluate this gene–drug interaction.[8,9]

Chapter Summary

As with other reduced-function alleles related to metabolism, the substrate, here SN-38, increases in patients who are carriers of the

UGT1A1*28 allele, resulting in potentially life-threatening adverse events. Patients who are homozygous for the UGT1A1*28 allele are especially at risk for toxicity. Genetic testing can help identify these patients and allow for the use of an appropriate dose of irinotecan.

Answers to Case Questions

1. A decrease in starting dose is recommended for patients who have been found to be homozygous for the UGT1A1*28 allele.
2. When first discussing the need for genetic testing, DT needs to be reassured that he is only being screened to determine his risk of toxicity relative to irinotecan. He will need to be assured that only genes involved in drug response are being screened and not his susceptibility to disease or anything else. The discussion should include how genetic screening can help to save his life, decrease side effects, and save him money. His genetic-screening results should be explained to him such that he understands that his therapeutic response to a regimen made specifically for him will improve as a result of determining his UGT1A1 expression. Furthermore, the decrease in the starting dose determined by his genetic screening will decrease his likelihood of suffering adverse events associated with irinotecan.

Review Questions

1. A patient who is homozygotic for the UGT1A1*28 allele would be predicted to have a higher plasma concentration of which of the following?
   a. Irinotecan
   b. SN-38
   c. SN-38G
   d. Irinotecan-G

2. The dose-limiting toxicities associated with irinotecan therapy include which of the following?
   a. Myelosuppression
   b. Diarrhea
   c. Nausea and vomiting
   d. a and b only
   e. a, b, and c

3. Which of the following is irinotecan's pharmacodynamic target?
   a. Dihydroxypyrimidine dehydrogenase
   b. Topoisomerase I
   c. Dihydrofolate reductase
   d. Thymidylate synthase

4. A patient who is homozygotic for the UGT1A1*28 allele would be predicted to have which of the following types of drug–gene interactions?

a. Pharmacodynamic

b. Pharmacokinetic

5. Which of the following patients would likely require the lowest starting dose of irinotecan?

a. A patient who is homozygotic for UGT1A1*28.

b. A patient who is heterozygotic for UGT1A1*28.

c. A chronic smoking patient who is heterozygotic for UGT1A1*28.

d. A chronic smoking patient who is homozygotic for UGT1A1*28.

References

1. Martinez-Balibrea E, Abad A, Martínez-Cardú A, et al. UGT1A and TYMS genetic variants predict toxicity and response of colorectal cancer patients treated with first-line irinotecan and fluorouracil combination therapy. Br J Cancer. 2010;103:581–589.

2. Ramesh M, Ahlawat P, Srinivas NR. Irinotecan and its metabolite, SN-38: review of bioanalytical methods and recent update from clinical pharmacology perspectives. Biomed Chromatogr. 2010;24:104–123.

3. de Jong MJA, Sparreboom A, Verweij J. The development of combination therapy involving camptothecins: a review of preclinical and early clinical studies. Cancer Treat Rev. 1998;24:205–220.

4. Gupta E, Lestingi TM, Mick R, Ramirez J, Vokes EE, Ratain MJ. Metabolic fate of irinotecan in humans: correlation of glucuronidation with diarrhea. Cancer Res. 1994;54:3723–3725.

5. Sugiyama Y, Kato Y, Chu X. Multiplicity of biliary excretion mechanisms for camptothecin derivative irinotecan (CPT-11), its metabolite SN-38, and its glucuronide: role of canalicular multispecific organic anion transporter and P-glycoprotein. Cancer Chemother Pharmacol. 1998;42(suppl):S44–S49.

6. van der Bol JM, Mathijssen RH, Loos WJ, et al. Cigarette smoking and irinotecan treatment: Pharmacokinetic interaction and effects on neutropenia. J Clin Oncol. 2007;25:2719–2726.

7. Benowitz NL. Cigarette smoking and the personalization of irinotecan therapy. J Clin Onc. 2007;25(19):2646–2647.

8. Swen JJ, Nijenhuis M, de Boer A, et al. Pharmacogenetics: From bench to byte—an update of guidelines. Clin Pharmacol Ther. 2011;89(5):662–673.

9. PharmGKB. Gene–drug pairs. Available at: www.pharmgkb.org/page/cpicGeneDrugPairs. Accessed July 29, 2012.

Chapter **9**

6-Mercaptopurine/ Azathioprine

LEARNING OBJECTIVES

Upon completion of this chapter, the student will be able to:

1. Recognize the various genotypes of thiopurine methyltransferase (TPMT) relative to 6-mercaptopurine metabolism.
2. Explain the appropriate use of genetic testing in an individual who is to receive 6-mercaptopurine.
3. Interpret and utilize genetic testing information relative to 6-mercaptopurine.

> Students need to understand the potential for a gene–drug interaction related to a drug metabolizing enzyme, recognizing that variation in a drug metabolizing enzyme can lead to severe toxicity and death with standard dosing of 6-mercaptopurine. A valid genetic test can indicate a patient's risk of toxicity due to decreased drug metabolism.

CASE QUESTIONS

Upon completion of this chapter, the student will be able to answer the following questions pertaining to the case of CP:

1. Based on CP's genetic constitution, would a standard dose of 6-mercaptopurine be warranted?
2. Is genetic testing required for all individuals who are to receive 6-mercaptopurine?

Key Terms	
genotype	The specific set of alleles inherited at a locus on a given gene.
pharmacodynamic	The relationship between drug exposure and pharmacologic response.
pharmacokinetic	The relationship of time and drug absorption, distribution, metabolism, and excretion.
prodrug	A drug that requires conversion to an active form.

Introduction

CP is a 10-year-old Caucasian male with a three-month history of general malaise, severe nosebleeds, frequent infections, and, more recently, swollen lymph nodes in the neck. Additionally, CP has been experiencing fever and bleeding of his gums (with and without brushing). CP is pale in appearance and complains of being "very tired."

The patient's family history includes an older sibling who was diagnosed with acute lymphocytic leukemia (ALL) at the age of 12 years. Physical exam, blood work, and a bone marrow biopsy indicate that CP has the same disease (ALL) as that diagnosed earlier in his older brother. CP undergoes successful chemotherapy, which results in remission of the disease. CP undergoes consolidation/intensification treatment along with central nervous system sanctuary therapy. At this time, maintenance therapy is considered. However, it is noted that CP's brother nearly died due to myelosuppression following the initiation of maintenance therapy with 6-mercaptopurine (6-MP) and methotrexate. The board-certified oncology pharmacist explains the benefits of genetic testing, especially in this setting. Therefore, prior to initiation of maintenance therapy with 6-MP, CP has genetic testing performed to evaluate the activity of thiopurine methyltransferase (TPMT), which is responsible for the metabolism of 6-MP.[1,2] With testing, it is noted that CP carries a TPMT variant allele, having the **genotype** *1/*3A.

Note that because approximately 90% of a dose of azathioprine is converted to 6-MP, this chapter will address 6-MP.

6-Mercaptopurine Pharmacodynamics

6-Mercaptopurine, which was first synthesized in the early 1950s, has been a long-standing ALL maintenance therapy in combination with methotrexate.[3–5] 6-Mercaptopurine, which is taken up by cells via nucleoside transporters, is an inactive **prodrug** that requires activation within the cell to eventually form the cytotoxic compound thio-deoxyguanosine triphosphate (TdGTP).[2,6,7] The incorporation of TdGTP into DNA inhibits the action of a number of enzymes relevant to replication and repair of DNA. Damage to DNA ensues, including single-strand breaks and other terminal events.[8,9]

6-Mercaptopurine Pharmacokinetics

The metabolic pathway of interest involves conversion of 6-MP to thioinosine monophosphate (TIMP) by hypoxanthine guanine phosphoribosyl transferase (HPRT1). Subsequently, TIMP is converted to thioxanthosine monophosphate (TXMP) via inositol monophosphate dehydrogenase (IMPDH), and then to thioguanosine monophosphate (TGMP) by guanosine monophosphate synthetase (GMPS). At this point, TGMP can go on to eventually form TdGTP, as stated earlier, eliciting a therapeutic effect, or TGMP can be metabolized by TPMT to form 6-methyl-thioguanine monophosphate (6-MeTGMP; **Figure 9-1**). Thus, competition occurs between the conversion of TGMP via the activation pathway to form TdGTP and the conversion of TGMP via the metabolic pathway to form 6-MeTGMP. An inverse relationship exists between TPMT activity and the formation of the active metabolites of 6-MP.

The polymorphic TPMT is the potential cause of severe, potentially life-threatening, myelosuppression. The wild-type TPMT (*1/*1) denotes normal metabolic function, and individuals with this genotype are dosed with the typical starting dose of 6-MP. Although there are more than 15 known TPMT alleles, the frequency of the nonfunctional alleles *2, *3A, *3B, *3C, and *4 are of concern when initiating therapy with 6-MP or azathioprine.[2,10] These variant

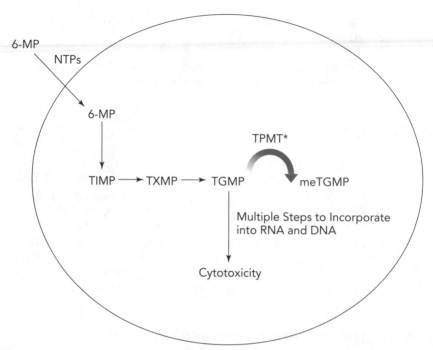

Figure 9-1 Following transport into cells via nucleoside transporters (NTPs), one metabolic step of interest is thioguanine monophosphate (TGMP) conversion via thiopurine methyltransferase (TPMT) to meTGMP. The polymorphisms seen with respect to TPMT* affect the potential toxicity of 6-mercaptopurine. TIMP = thioinosine monophosphate, TXMP = thioxanthosine monophophate.

alleles constitute greater than 90% of the nonfunctioning alleles, with approximately 1 in 178 to 1 in 3,736 patients being homozygous for a nonfunctioning allele. These individuals would be at greater risk of life-threatening 6-MP–induced toxicity. Additionally, approximately 3% to 14% of individuals are heterozygous for one nonfunctional allele, thus imparting a risk of moderate toxicity with the use of standard doses of 6-MP. Additionally, a number of rare alleles, including *6, *9, *10, *11, *12,*13, *16, *17, and *18, appear to impart a reduced-function TPMT. **Table 9-1** presents information on the frequency of alleles in various populations.

Individuals who are heterozygous with one normal-function allele and one nonfunctional allele require a lower dose of 6-MP to avoid toxicity. This is especially important when treatment is for a malignant disease, such as ALL, for which higher starting doses are used as compared to doses used for nonmalignant diseases. In this case, the dose of 6-MP should be 30% to 70% of the usual dose.[10–12] For patients who are homozygous for nonfunctional alleles, the dose should be reduced by 10-fold and be administered less frequently (typically three times weekly as compared to once

Table 9-1

Average Frequencies of the *1 TPMT Allele and Highest Frequency of a Given Nonfunctional Allele in Selected Populations[a]

Allele	Caucasian	Mediterranean	South American	African	Middle Eastern	Mexican	Asian	Southwest Asian
Frequencies of the *1 allele in selected populations.								
*1	0.95671	0.96081	0.95233	0.94284	0.96987	0.925	0.98364	0.97837
Highest frequency of nonfunctioning allele (*3A, *3C) in selected populations.								
*3A	0.0354	0.0254	0.0287		0.0114	0.0533		
*3C				0.048			0.0157	0.0133

[a] The *2, *3B, and *4 alleles occur in the above populations at lower frequencies than noted for the *3A and *3C alleles.

Source: Adapted from Relling MV, Pui CH, Cheng C, Evans WE. Thiopurine methyltransferase in acute lymphoblastic leukemia. *Blood.* 2006;107:843–844. Supplemental information available at http://pharmgkb.org/drug/PA450379#tabview =tab0&subtab=31.

daily).[10–12] Failure to adjust the dose of 6-MP downward for patients with loss-of-function alleles can result in fatal toxicity. Here, a **pharmacokinetic** alteration (metabolism) results in toxicity (**pharmacodynamic** end point). Dosing guidelines for 6-MP and other thiopurines have been developed by the Clinical Pharmacogenetics Implementation Consortium.[10]

Chapter Summary

Patients who are to receive 6-MP may be at risk of severe toxicity due to the potential of having reduced or loss-of-function TPMT. Although genetic testing is not currently required prior to the use of 6-MP, it is recommended that such testing be performed. Although patients who are homozygous for reduced or loss-of-function TPMT alleles are at risk of toxicity, patients who are heterozygotes are also at risk and require downward dosage adjustment.

Answers to Case Questions

1. The TPMT*1/*3A genotype reveals that CP has one loss-of-function allele (*3A). Therefore, CP would require a lower dose of 30% to 70% of the normal full starting dose. The dose can be adjusted based on the level of myelosuppression.
2. Currently, genotyping for TPMT is recommended but not mandatory. However, in CP's case there is a clear rationale

for genetic screening. It is recommended that individuals who are to receive 6-MP (or other thiopurines) have their TPMT genotype determined.[10]

Review Questions

1. A patient with ALL is to receive 6-MP for maintenance therapy. The patient's genotype is determined, relative to TPMT activity, and the results identify that the patient's genotype is *1/*3C. Based on this information, which of the following is correct?
   a. The patient should receive the usual dose of 6-MP.
   b. The patient should receive a dose that is 30% to 70% of the usual dose.
   c. The patient should receive a dose that is reduced 10-fold as compared to the usual dose.
   d. The patient should receive an increased dose of 6-MP relative to the usual dose.

2. With respect to TPMT and genotype, which of the following patients would be *least* likely to experience severe myelosuppression due to 6-MP administration?
   a. *1/*1
   b. *1/*3C
   c. *2/*3A
   d. *3A/*3C

3. The interaction between the genetic makeup of an individual relative to TPMT and myelosuppression with 6-MP dosing is a result of which of the following?
   a. A gene–pharmacokinetic interaction
   b. A gene–toxicokinetic interaction
   c. A gene–pharmacokinetic–pharmacodynamic interaction
   d. An idiosyncratic reaction (one of unknown origin)

4. 6-Mercaptopurine and azathioprine cannot be used in patients with two loss-of-function alleles relative to TPMT.
   a. True
   b. False

5. Because azathioprine is a prodrug of 6-mercaptopurine, similar dosing considerations need to be considered in patients who are either heterozygous (wild-type and nonfunctional alleles) or homozygous for deficient alleles.
   a. True
   b. False

References

1. McLeod HL, Krynetski EY, Relling MV, Evans WE. Genetic polymorphism of thiopurine methyltransferase and its clinical relevance for childhood acute lymphocytic leukemia. *Leukemia.* 2000;14:567–572.

2. Sahasranaman S, Howard D, Roy S. Clinical pharmacology and pharmacogenetics of thiopurines. *Eur J Clin Pharmacol.* 2008;64:753–767.

3. Elion GB, Hitchings GH, Vanderwerff H. Antagonists of nucleic acid derivatives: VI. Purines. *J Biol Chem.* 1951;192(2):505–518.

4. Hitchings GH, Elion GB. The chemistry and biochemistry of purine analogs. *Ann NY Acad Sci.* 1954;60(2):195–199.

5. Schmiegelow K, Schrøder H, Schmiegelow M. Methotrexate and 6-mercaptopurine maintenance therapy for childhood acute lymphoblastic leukemia: dose adjustments by white cell counts or by pharmacokinetic parameters? *Cancer Chemother Pharmacol.* 1994;34(3):209–15.

6. Salser JS, Balis ME. The mechanism of action of 6-mercaptopurine. *Cancer Res.* 1965;25:539–543.

7. Fotoohi AK, Lindqvist M, Peterson C, Albertioni F. Involvement of the concentrative nucleoside transporter 3 and equilibrative nucleoside transporter 2 in the resistance of T-lymphoblastic cell lines to thiopurines. *Biochem Biophys Res Commun.* 2006; 343(1):208–215.

8. Swann PF, Waters TR, Moulton DC, et al. Role of postreplicative DNA mismatch repair in the cytotoxic action of thioguanine. *Science.* 1996;273(5278): 1109–1111.

9. Lennard L. The clinical pharmacology of 6-mercaptopurine. *Eur J Clin Pharmacol.* 1992;43(4):329–339.

10. Relling MV, Gardner EE, Sandborn WJ, et al. Clinical Pharmacogenetics Implementation Consortium guidelines for thiopurine methyltransferase genotype and thiopurine dosing. *Clin Pharmacol Ther.* 2011;89(3):387–391.

11. Evans WE, Horner M, Chu YQ, Kalwinsky D, Roberts WM. Altered mercaptopurine metabolism, toxic effects, and dosage requirement in a thiopurine methyltransferase-deficient child with acute lymphocytic leukemia. *J Pediatr.* 1991;119:985–989.

12. Relling MV, Pui CH, Cheng C, Evans WE. Thiopurine methyltransferase in acute lymphoblastic leukemia. *Blood.* 2006;107:843–844.

Chapter 10

Warfarin

LEARNING OBJECTIVES

Upon completion of this chapter, the student will be able to:

1. Recognize the various genotypes of cytochrome P450-2C9 (CYP2C9) relative to warfarin metabolism.
2. Recognize the various haplotypes of vitamin K epoxide reductase (VKORC1) relative to warfarin activity.
3. Explain the appropriate use of genetic testing in an individual who is to receive warfarin.
4. Interpret and utilize genetic testing information relative to warfarin.

The student should understand the influence of genetic variation in a drug metabolism enzyme and a drug target protein. The student also should recognize that more than one valid genetic test is needed to be able to appropriately predict and evaluate a given patient's response to warfarin.

CASE QUESTIONS

Upon completion of this chapter, the student will be able to answer the following questions pertaining to the case of LK:

1. Based on LK's genetic constitution, would a standard dose of warfarin be warranted?
2. Why did the pharmacist point out that although determination of the dosing regimen of warfarin would be aided by genetic evaluation, the clinical outcome of warfarin use based on genetic information is not known?

Key Terms	
CYP; CYP450	The cytochrome P450 oxidative metabolic enzyme superfamily.
haplotype	Regions of DNA containing multiple single nucleotide polymorphisms (SNPs).
pharmacodynamics (PD)	The relationship between drug exposure and pharmacologic response.
pharmacokinetics (PK)	The relationship of time and drug absorption, distribution, metabolism, and excretion.
pharmacogenetics (PGt)	The study of a gene involved in response to a drug.
reference SNP number (refSNP; rs#)	A number that is a unique and consistent identifier of a given SNP.

Key Equations	
$D_M = C_{ss} \cdot CL$	The maintenance dose related to the desired steady-state concentration and clearance.
$E = E_0 - \dfrac{(E_{max})(C^{\gamma})}{EC_{50}^{\gamma} + C^{\gamma}}$	The effect related to the baseline effect, the maximal effect, and drug concentration and inversely related to drug concentration eliciting a half-maximal response and the drug concentration.

Introduction

LK is a 57-year-old Caucasian male with a 19-year history of hypertension (stage 1; 148/92 mm Hg). He sees his family practice physician with complaints of shortness of breath with normal activity, lack of energy, and a sensation of his heart "racing" in his chest. An ECG is performed, and LK is diagnosed with atrial fibrillation, with a heart rate of 147 beats per minute (bpm) at rest. LK is referred to a cardiologist. The completion and review of a 48-hour Holter monitor study confirms this diagnosis.

LK is a writer for a national baseball website. He is sedentary much of the day because he works at his computer. He is overweight and is taking the following medications: atorvastatin 10 mg each morning, aspirin 81 mg each morning, hydrochlorothiazide 25 mg each morning, and a daily multivitamin. LK does not smoke, nor does he drink alcohol.

Included in LK's treatment plan is the use of the anticoagulant warfarin to reduce blood clot formation and the risk of cerebral vascular accident (CVA). LK is referred to the pharmacy department's "anticoag clinic," where specific attention is paid to optimizing therapy with warfarin. The treatment goal for LK is the prevention of blood clots while avoiding bleeding episodes, which are a significant risk of warfarin therapy. As part of the clinic's approach to warfarin therapy, patients are asked to have their genetic information screened for variants of cytochrome P450-2C9 (**CYP**2C9). This is the major metabolic enzyme responsible for metabolism of the more active S-enantiomer of warfarin. The clinic also employs genetic testing of vitamin K epoxide reductase subunit 1 (VKORC1), which is responsible for vitamin K reduction, leading to activation of blood clotting factors.[1] With testing, it is noted that LK carries a CYP2C9 allelic variant, having the genotype *2/*2. It also is noted that LK has the AG genotype for VKORC1 related to the *2 haplotype.

The pharmacist explains that LK's genetic constitution requires him to receive a lower dose of warfarin as compared to the average individual. It also is explained to LK that the genetic information will be used to design a therapeutic regimen that will hopefully optimize anticoagulation while avoiding bleeding events. The goal is to rapidly achieve an appropriate international normalized ratio (INR) with warfarin. The pharmacist explains that although there is preliminary research showing that genotype-guided warfarin prescribing helps move patients into a therapeutic INR range sooner, the true outcome of the genetically guided therapy cannot be predicted at this time.

Warfarin, a mainstay in anticoagulation therapy, is a very difficult drug to dose correctly. The drug's **pharmacokinetics (PK)** are marked by stereochemical differences, genetic variation in metabolism, and dietary influences, among other variables. Warfarin's **pharmacodynamics (PD)** are examined in the context of the intricate coagulation system and the genetic variation that further complicate dosing.[2]

Warfarin Pharmacodynamics

Genetic variability relative to dosage requirements for patients on warfarin includes a pharmacodynamic component. Vitamin K epoxide reductase subunit 1 is responsible for reducing vitamin K 2,3-epoxide back to the active form of vitamin K after the activation of clotting factors (see **Figure 10-1**). This active form of vitamin K is needed for carboxylation of glutamic acid residues in some clotting proteins. The specific clotting proteins (II, VII, IX, and X) are referred to as vitamin K–dependent clotting factors. Thus, VKORC1 "recycles" vitamin K, which aids in the production of active clotting factors. Warfarin is effective as an anticoagulant because it inhibits VKORC1, resulting in decreased active vitamin K and inactive vitamin K–dependent clotting factors. It appears from numerous reports that the genotype of VKORC1 is of greater significance in determining the warfarin maintenance dose than is the CYP2C9 genotype.[3–5]

Four significant **haplotypes**—regions of the DNA with multiple SNPs—that are related to variations in VKORC1 have been identified. These haplotypes are termed VKORC1*1, *2, *3, and *4, with VKORC1*1 being considered the wild-type, exhibiting normal protein activity.[6] The *2 variant (including rs9923231), also known as haplotype group A, designates an individual who produces lower amounts of VKORC1 and is more sensitive to warfarin. Such a patient would require a lower warfarin dose for therapeutic efficacy.[6,7] The *2 variant is most prevalent in the Asian population (~90%) and among Caucasians (~40%); it is present in only 11% of African Americans. The basis for this variant is an adenine (A) at position 3673 and a thymine (T) at position 6484 of the haplotype.[6] VKORC1*3 and VKORC1*4 are similar, being differentiated mainly by a SNP at position 9041; individuals homozygous for the *3 or *4 variant require a relative higher dose of warfarin.[6] The *3 and *4 variants are seen in approximately 20% and 10%, respectively, of African Americans, and the *4 variant is observed in 20% of individuals of European descent.

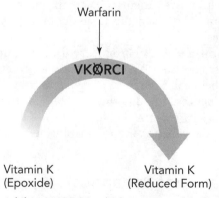

Figure 10-1 Warfarin inhibits VKORC1, which is responsible for producing the reduced form of vitamin K, which is essential for the formation of functional clotting factors (II, VII, IX, and X). In the face of reduced VKORC1, less warfarin is required to elicit an effect.

Warfarin Pharmacokinetics

Commercially available warfarin products are a 50:50 racemic mixture with different metabolic pathways for the R-warfarin and S-warfarin enantiomers. The R-warfarin isomer is metabolized by CYP1A1, CYP1A2, CYP2C19, and CYP3A4 as well as other non-CYP enzymes. The S-warfarin isomer is approximately five times more potent than its R-warfarin counterpart and is almost exclusively metabolized by CYP2C9, although CYP2C8, CYP2C18, and CYP2C19 play minor, negligible roles in its elimination (see **Figure 10-2**).[8–10] It is the genetic variation in VKORC1 and CYP2C9 that is largely responsible for the varied dose requirements among patients.

The large variability in the metabolism of S-warfarin has been attributed to the single nucleotide polymorphisms (SNPs) of CYP2C9.[11] The gene encoding for the CYP2C9 enzyme is located on chromo-

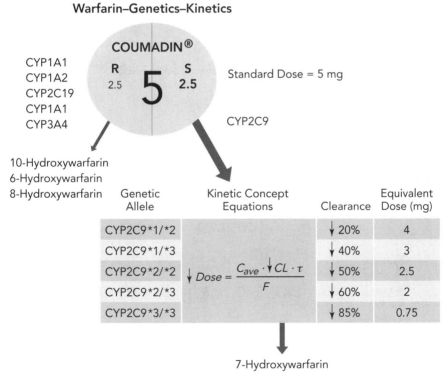

Warfarin–Genetics–Kinetics

Genetic Allele	Kinetic Concept Equations	Clearance	Equivalent Dose (mg)
CYP2C9*1/*2		↓20%	4
CYP2C9*1/*3		↓40%	3
CYP2C9*2/*2	$\downarrow Dose = \dfrac{C_{ave} \cdot \downarrow CL \cdot \tau}{F}$	↓50%	2.5
CYP2C9*2/*3		↓60%	2
CYP2C9*3/*3		↓85%	0.75

7-Hydroxywarfarin

Figure 10-2 The racemic (50/50) R/S warfarin is metabolized by various cytochrome P450 enzymes, with CYP2C9 being of major importance as it metabolizes the more potent S form of the drug. Reduced function CYP2C9 alleles (*2, *3) result in a decreased clearance of the S form of warfarin and thus patients with reduced functioning CYP2C9 require lower doses of the drug.

some 10, and numerous SNPs related to this gene have been identified, with the majority producing malfunctioning proteins. Evaluation
of CYP2C9 in 192 European American patients receiving warfarin
detected 132 SNPs, of which eight were nonsynonymous SNPs
found in the coding region.[12] The SNPs code for a number of alleles,
including CYP2C9*2, *3, *9, *11, and *12. Of these, CYP2C9*2 and
CYP2C9*3 were represented at a significant frequency (> 1%) of
11% and 6%, respectively (see **Figure 10-3**).[12] Both of these alleles
were associated with a statistically significant lower warfarin dosage
requirement.[12]

Similar to the above findings, CYP2C9 allele frequencies were studied
in two patient groups.[13] One group consisted of 177 Caucasian patients
and 12 additional patients of various ethnicities. The *2 allele was present
in 11.6% of the Caucasian patients, and the *3 allele was present in 6.9% of
the Caucasians patients. The second group (a comparison control group)

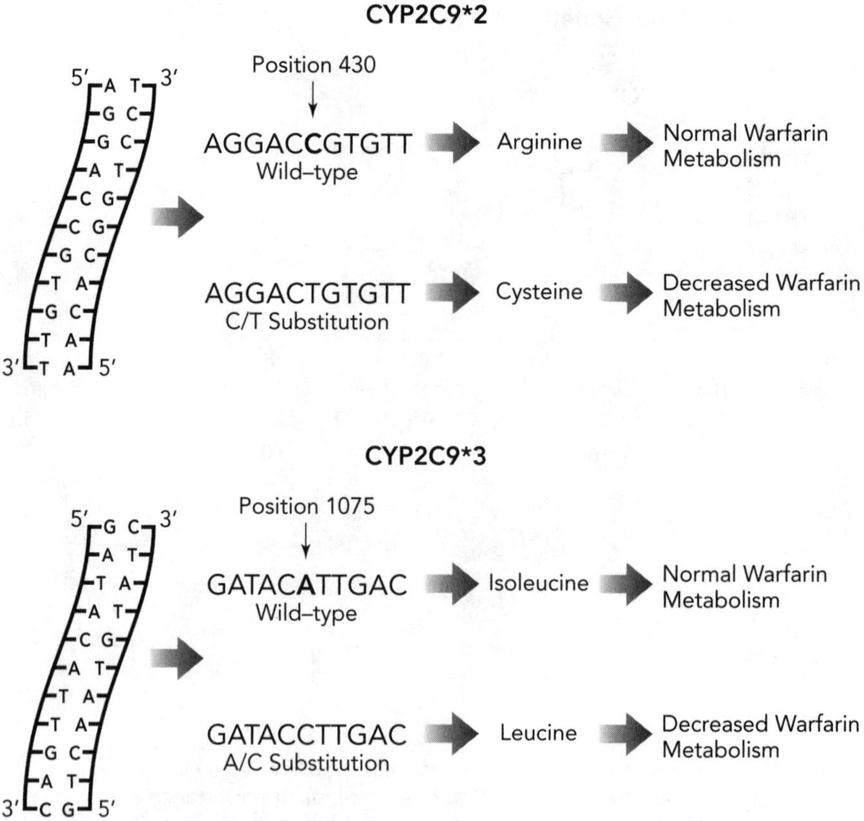

Figure 10-3 Example of CYP2C9 SNPs resulting in decreased metabolic function
relative to warfarin metabolism.
Note: On the continuous DNA strands, the first two bases are the last two of a
codon, with subsequent codons following.

consisted of Caucasians (n = 87), Asians (n = 44), and African Americans (n = 47). The *2 allele was found in 15.5% of the Caucasian patients and in 1.1% of the combined Asian and African American cohorts. The *3 allele was seen in 6.9% of Caucasian patients, but was only present in 1.7% of Asian/African American patients.[13] These reported allele frequencies for CYP2C9*2 and CYP2C9*3 in the first group are comparable to earlier reports in a similar population with values of 12.2% and 7.9%, respectively.[14] Patients in this evaluation expressing the *1/*3, *2/*2, *2/*3, and the *3/*3 genotypes had a statistically significant lower warfarin dosage requirement, with the *2/*3 and *3/*3 individuals requiring the lowest doses.[13] **Table 10-1** presents examples of the known CYP2C9 SNPs with relevance to enzyme activity. The **reference SNP numbers** are provided (rs#). These numbers are unique and consistent identifiers of the given SNP.

The identified SNPs resulting in various CYP2C9 alleles and altered enzyme metabolic capacity have been a major component of genotype-guided warfarin therapy. However, an association between another CYP enzyme and warfarin dose requirement has been identified. A SNP in the CYP4F2 gene has been associated with as much as a 25% variance in the daily dose of warfarin.[15] The altered warfarin dosing requirements with variants of CYP4F2 are related to decreasing vitamin K availability via vitamin K_1 oxidation, not the metabolism of warfarin (i.e., a pharmacodynamic interaction).[16,17] Subsequently, a genome-wide study confirmed that CYP4F2 SNPs accounted for 0.5 mg/day differences in the warfarin dosage requirement.[18] Clearly, more research is needed to look at this enzyme's influence relative to genotype-guided warfarin therapy.

Combining the CYP2C9 and VKORC1 information allows the use of the FDA-approved dosing guideline table presented in the warfarin package labeling (see **Table 10-2**).[20]

Table 10-1			
Representative Single Nucleotide Polymorphisms for CYP2C9			
Allele	**Nucleotide Change**	**SNP rs#[a]**	**Enzyme Activity**
CYP2C9*1[b]			Normal
CYP2C9*2[b]	430C>T	rs1799853	Reduced
CYP2C9*3[b]	1075A>C	rs1057910	Reduced
CYP2C9*4	1076T>C	rs56165452	Reduced
CYP2C9*5	1080C>G	rs28371686	Reduced

[a] A number that is a unique and consistent identifier of a given SNP.
[b] Seen in populations at significant frequencies (> 1%).

Genetic–Kinetic Interface: Warfarin Dosing and CYP2C9

A patient is diagnosed with proximal deep venous thrombosis, having experienced right leg calf pain following knee replacement surgery. The patient is to be started on warfarin and is to be maintained on the drug for six months. In consultation with a pharmacist at the anticoagulation clinic, the patient's physician orders genetic testing to determine the patient's CYP2C9 and VKORC1 genotype. The results indicate that the patient has a variant CYP2C9 allele with the genotype being CYP2C9*1/*3. However, the VKORC1 results are delayed. The patient's maintenance dose is determined to be 3 mg per day.

The patient is heterozygous for a reduced-function allele (*1/*3), which indicates the need for a lower-than-normal maintenance warfarin dose. Therefore, the patient receives a maintenance dose of 3 mg per day as compared to 5 mg per day. The decreased-functioning CYP2C9 enzyme results in decreased clearance of warfarin. Because clearance is utilized in calculating the maintenance dose (D_M), the resultant dosing requirements reflects the patient's CYP2C9*1/*3 status:

$$\downarrow D_M = C_{SS} \cdot \downarrow CL$$

Although it is not the standard of practice to monitor the concentration of warfarin (C_{ss}), the concentration is a result of a given dose. Understanding that the clearance of warfarin is decreased in this individual, and desiring a similar average warfarin concentration to that which would be produced by the "average" dose, it is understood that the dose needs to be reduced. The goal here is to have the patient's INR within the therapeutic range (2.0–3.0) to achieve anticoagulation.

Genetic–Kinetic–Dynamic Interface: Warfarin Dosing, CYP2C9, and VKORC1

An individual receives his genome results based on the saliva sample he provided to a direct-to-consumer "personal genome" company. Because the individual is a pharmacist and is interested in the drug response results, he looks at the information provided regarding warfarin. The results state that he has "increased sensitivity" to warfarin. With some investigation, he sees the following information: CYP2C9*1/*1, VKORC1 –1639/3673 AA

The CYP2C9*1/*1 result means that he has the normal-function metabolizing enzyme. This allelic designation is related to pharmacokinetics, because the clearance (which determines the maintenance dose) would be considered to be average. Based on this information alone, if he were to require warfarin therapy the average dose would be sufficient.

However, with respect to the pharmacogenetic–pharmacodynamic relationship, the VKORC1 –1639/3673 AA designation (also named rs9923231), which is another term that refers to the VKORC1*2 haplotype, indicates that if he were to receive warfarin he would need a lower-than-average dose. The following inhibitory E_{max} (baseline subtraction) model best describes the anticoagulation effect, with the VKORC1 genotype being related to warfarin sensitivity:

$$E = E_0 - \frac{(E_{max})(C^\gamma)}{EC_{50}^\gamma + C^\gamma}$$

Here, the –1639/3673 AA genotype results in the lowest EC_{50} value, indicating the increased sensitivity to warfarin.[19]

Table 10-2

Range of Expected Therapeutic Warfarin Maintenance Doses Based on CYP2C9 and VKORC1 Genotypes

VKORC1 Genotypes	Cytochrome P450 CYP2C9 Genotypes					
	*1/*1	*1/*2	*1/*3	*2/*2	*2/*3	*3/*3
G/G	5–7 mg/d	5–7 mg/d	3–4 mg/d	3–4 mg/d	3–4 mg/d	0.5–2 mg/d
A/G	5–7 mg/d	3–4 mg/d	3–4 mg/d	3–4 mg/d	0.5–2 mg/d	0.5–2 mg/d
A/A	3–4 mg/d	3–4 mg/d	0.5–2 mg/d	0.5–2 mg/d	0.5–2 mg/d	0.5–2 mg/d

Source: Coumadin tablets (warfarin sodium tablets, USP) crystalline Coumadin for injection (warfarin sodium for injection, USP). Package labeling can be found at http://packageinserts.bms.com/ pi/pi_coumadin.pdf. Accessed October 17, 2011.

Chapter Summary

Millions of warfarin prescriptions are filled in the United States each year.[21] Historically, the approach to initial warfarin dosing has been based solely on trial and error, where doses are adjusted frequently until the patient is stable with an acceptable therapeutic INR, generally between 2.0–3.0. The Clinical Pharmacogenetic Implementation Consortium warfarin dosing guidelines were published in 2011 and provide a clear approach to the application of **pharmacogenetic (PGt)** information.[17] The advent of PGt dosing of warfarin has been shown to improve initial dosing; however, further experience and documentation of PGt dosing is needed.[22]

Answers to Case Questions

1. The CYP2C9*2/*2 genotype is associated with a lower required dose of warfarin. Additionally, the VKORC1 AG genotype is also related to a lower dose requirement, such that the dose requirement of warfarin in a patient with these genotypes is approximately half the average dose.
2. Although one study has shown that the use of genotype-guided warfarin dosing puts an individual into the INR therapeutic range sooner and decreases the incidence of minor bleeds, further studies are needed in larger populations to confirm these findings.

Review Questions

1. Which of the following CYP2C9 alleles are considered reduced-function alleles?
   a. *2
   b. *1
   c. *3
   d. Both a and c
   e. a, b, and c

2. The interaction between the VKORC1 gene and warfarin is considered to be a:
   a. pharmacokinetic interaction.
   b. pharmacogenetic interaction.
   c. pharmacogenomic interaction.
   d. pharmacodynamic interaction.
   e. non-interaction.

3. Consider the following table, as presented in the warfarin package labeling:

VKORC1 Genotypes	Cytochrome P450 CYP2C9 Genotypes					
	*1/*1	*1/*2	*1/*3	*2/*2	*2/*3	*3/*3
G/G	5–7 mg/d	5–7 mg/d	3–4 mg/d	3–4 mg/d	3–4 mg/d	0.5–2 mg/d
A/G	5–7 mg/d	3–4 mg/d	3–4 mg/d	3–4 mg/d	0.5–2 mg/d	0.5–2 mg/d
A/A	3–4 mg/d	3–4 mg/d	0.5–2 mg/d	0.5–2 mg/d	0.5–2 mg/d	0.5–2 mg/d

Source: Coumadin tablets (warfarin sodium tablets, USP) crystalline Coumadin for injection (warfarin sodium for injection, USP). Package labeling can be found at http://packageinserts.bms.com/ pi/pi_coumadin.pdf. Accessed October 17, 2011.

A patient has the genotypes of *1/*3 and A/G for CYP2C9 and VKORC1, respectively. What initial maintenance dose would you recommend for this patient?
a. 5 mg daily
b. 3 mg daily
c. 7 mg daily
d. 2 mg daily
e. 6 mg daily

4. An individual with a CYP2C9*2/*3 genotype would require a lower maintenance dose of warfarin because the drug's _____ is decreased.
a. clearance
b. volume of distribution
c. half-life
d. absorption rate
e. renal elimination

5. Which of the following CYP2C9 reduced-function alleles is seen in the highest percentage of patients across ethnicities?
a. *3
b. *5
c. *11
d. *8
e. *2

References

1. Limdi NA, Veenstra DL. Warfarin pharmacogenomics. *Pharmacotherapy.* 2008;28(9):1084–1097.
2. Glurich I, Burmester JK, Caldwell MD. Understanding the pharmacogenetic approach to warfarin dosing. *Heart Fail Rev.* 2010;15:239–248.
3. Yin T, Miyata T. Warfarin dose and the pharmacogenomics of CYP2C9 and VKORC1-rationale and perspectives. *Thromb Res.* 2007;120:1–10.
4. Wen MS, Lee M, Chen JJ, et al. Prospective study of warfarin dosage requirements based on CYP2C9 and VKORC1 genotypes. *Clin Pharmacol Ther.* 2008;84:83–89.

5. Wedalius M, Chen LY, Lindh JD, et al. The largest prospective warfarin-treated cohort supports genetic forecasting. Blood. 2009;113:784–792.

6. Geisen C, Watzka M, Sittinger K, et al. VKORC1 haplotypes and their impact on the inter-individual and inter-ethnical variability of oral anticoagulation. Thromb Haemost. 2005;94:773–779.

7. Rieder MJ, Reiner AP, Gage BF, et al. Effect of VKORC1 haplotypes on transcriptional regulation and warfarin dose. N Engl J Med. 2005;352(22):2285–2293.

8. Kaminsky LS, Zhang. Human P450 metabolism of warfarin. Pharmacol Ther. 1997;73:67–74.

9. Rettie AE, Korzekwa KR, Kunze KL, et al. Hydroxylation of warfarin by human cDNA-expressed cytochrome P-450: A role for P-4502C9 in the etiology of (S)-warfarin-drug interactions. Chem Res Tox. 1992;5:54–59.

10. Yamazaki H, Shimada T. Human liver cytochrome P450 enzymes involved in the 7-hydroxylation of R and S warfarin enantiomers. Biochem Pharmacol. 1997;54:1195–1203.

11. Caraco Y, Muszkat M, Wood AJJ. Phenytoin metabolic ratio, a putative probe of CYP2C9 activity in-vivo. Pharmacogenetics. 2001;11:587–596.

12. Veenstra DL, Blough DK, Higashi MK, et al. CYP2C9 haplotype structure in European American warfarin patients and association with clinical outcomes. Clin Pharmacol Ther. 2005;77:353–364.

13. Moridani M, Fu L, Selby R, et al. Frequency of CYP2C9 polymorphisms affecting warfarin metabolism in a large anticoagulant clinic cohort. Clin Biochem. 2006;39:606–612.

14. Sanderson S, Emery J, Higgins J. CYP2C9 gene variations, drug dose, and bleeding risk in warfarin-treated patients: A HuGEnet systematic review and meta-analysis. Genet Med. 2005;7:97–104.

15. Caldwell MD, Awad T, Johnson JA, et al. CYP4F2 genetic variant alters required warfarin dose. Blood. 2008;111:4106–4112.

16. McDonald MG, Rieder MJ, Nakano M, Hsia CK, Rettie AE. CYP4F2 is a Vitamin K^1 oxidase: An explanation for altered warfarin dose in carriers of the V433M variant. Mol Pharmacol. 2009;75(6):1337–1346.

17. Johnson JA, Gong L, Whirl-Carrillo M, et al. Clinical Pharmacogenetics Implementation Consortium Guidelines for CYP2C9 and VKORC1 genotypes and warfarin dosing. Clin Pharmacol Ther. 2011;90(4):625–629.

18. Cooper GM, Johnson JA, Langaee TY, et al. A genome-wide scan for common genetic variants with a large influence on warfarin maintenance dose. Blood. 2008;112:1022–1027.

19. Hamberg AK, Dahl ML, Barban M, et al. A PK-PD model for predicting the impact of age, CYP2C9, and VKORC1 genotype on individualization of warfarin therapy. Clin Pharmacol Ther. 2007;81(4):529–538.

20. Coumadin tablets (warfarin sodium tablets, USP) crystalline Coumadin for injection (warfarin sodium for injection, USP). Package labeling available at: http://packageinserts.bms.com/pi/pi_coumadin.pdf. Accessed October 17, 2011.

21. Wysowski DK, Nourjah P, Swartz L. Bleeding complications with warfarin use a prevalent adverse effect resulting in regulatory action. Arch Intern Med. 2007;167:1414–1419.

22. Curaco Y, Blotnick S, Muszkat M. CYP2C9 genotype-guided warfarin prescribing enhances the efficacy and safety of anticoagulation: A prospective randomized controlled study. Clin Pharmacol Ther. 2008;83(3):460–470.

The Breadth of Personalized Medicine

Section IV introduces topics that constitute the breadth of personalized medicine. From the cost of whole-genome sequencing to the ethics of personalized medicine, these subjects represent some important aspects beyond the science. Additionally, a brief discussion of pharmacogenetics/pharmacogenomics resources is presented.

Chapter 11

The Breadth of Personalized Medicine

LEARNING OBJECTIVES

Upon completion of this chapter, the student will be able to:

1. Describe the evolution of DNA sequencing technology relative to cost of sequencing an entire genome (i.e., whole-genome sequencing).
2. Describe the need for education of healthcare providers, health professions students, and the general public with regard to personalized medicine.
3. Recognize available pharmacogenomics resources.
4. Recognize other technologies, beyond sequencing, that will impact personalized medicine.
5. Describe in broad terms the ethical and legal issues of personalized medicine.

> The student must understand that many factors will influence the use of pharmacogenetics/pharmacogenomics. From technology at the point of care to legal and ethical issues and education, clinical application of pharmacogenetics/pharmacogenomics will only become

widespread once these factors and others have been considered and acted upon.

Note that in this chapter we will use the term *pharmacogenomics* to encompass both pharmacogenetics and pharmacogenomics in our discussion of personalized medicine.

Key Terms	
Genetic Information Nondiscrimination Act (GINA)	Act by Congress that prohibits discrimination of an individual by health insurers and employers based on the individual's genetic information.
Health Insurance Portability and Accountability Act (HIPAA)	Act by Congress that allows individuals to keep their health insurance when they change or lose their job; decreases healthcare fraud and abuse; requires medical information confidentiality; and regulates industry standards related to medical billing and other processes.
Health Information Technology for Economic and Clinical Health Act (HITECH)	Part of the 2009 Recovery and Reinvestment Act mandating the use of electronic health records, primarily by physicians and hospitals.
pharmacogenetics (PGt)	The study of a gene involved in response to a drug.
pharmacogenomics (PGx)	The study of all genes in the genome involved in response to a drug.
single nucleotide polymorphism (SNP)	A variant DNA sequence in which a single nucleotide has been replaced by another such base.

Introduction

The science of **pharmacogenomics (PGx)**, when interfaced with pharmacokinetics and pharmacodynamics, is poised to revolutionize clinical therapeutics. Whether for specific drugs or general therapeutic decision making, the influence of PGx will be far reaching, impacting therapies and dosages, with the promise of improving therapeutic outcomes and decreasing adverse events.

It has been the lightning-speed improvements in efficiency in genome sequencing that has brought PGx to the clinical realm. With testing soon becoming available at costs similar to other laboratory test, the utility of genome sequencing may be realized.

With genome sequencing becoming more available, other issues come into play, such as education, whereby "the masses" of healthcare professionals and healthcare professions students will need to be educated on the appropriate interpretation and application of PGx test results.

Additionally, ethical, legal, and social issues will be brought to the forefront as more and more personal genetic data will be generated as whole-genome sequencing becomes standard. Healthcare professionals, insurers, employers, and society at large will have to learn how to handle and utilize this information in the light of expanded government regulation.

All of the above issues impact the use of genetic information and, in fact, will determine the scope of the use of the data, which will, in turn, determine how rapidly PGx becomes a standard of practice rather than a secluded, relatively infrequently used approach.

The Cost of Sequencing a Genome

As is the case with most technologies, the cost of a given technology and related ancillary items decreases with time. This is the case with whole-genome sequencing technologies. In 2001, the cost of whole-genome sequencing using the dideoxy ("Sanger") method was just under 100 million dollars ($95,263,072).[1,2] By January of 2005, the cost had dropped to $17.5 million, and as new second-generation sequencing technologies emerged the cost for whole-genome sequencing fell to just over $1.3 million by April of 2008. The rate of decline in the cost of whole-genome sequencing then accelerated, with the estimated cost being under $8,000 by January of 2012 (see **Figure 11-1**).[2,3] The cost will not stop at $8,000 because technology companies are continuing to explore next-generation sequencing methods, such as those that employ nanotechnology,

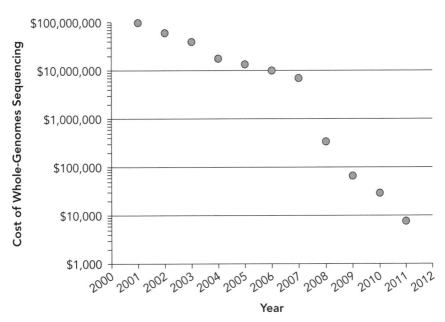

Figure 11-1 The cost of sequencing a complete (whole) genome has continued to decline, first following Moore's law (i.e., doubling capacity every 2 years) but then accelerating to a faster-paced reduction with the advent of new technologies starting in about 2008.

whereby DNA base pairs are read as they pass through nanopores.[4] These newer approaches increase efficiency, with more bases being read in a shorter amount of time, meaning whole genomes can be read within a day, if not hours. An ultimate goal is to have an accurate, reproducible method for sequencing at a cost of $1,000 or less. The actual utility cost will be higher because expertise is needed to interpret and apply the information provided by sequencing.

As the cost of genetic testing, here with regard specifically for drug therapy, continues to decrease, a broader population of clinicians will utilize the information in therapeutic decision making. Certainly as standards of care change the clinician will be obligated to incorporate PGx into practice or potentially face litigation.

Partial-genome testing has been underway for years, with direct-to-consumer companies providing information on **single nucleotide polymorphisms (SNPs)** of interest. For instance, one company offers "personal genome services" for as little as $299, providing information on more than 950,000 SNPs. Although this is not complete or whole-genome sequencing, the service does provide an immense amount of data directly to the consumer. This raises a number of issues, including those of data storage and handling; education and interpretation of data; and ethical, legal, and social considerations.

Although genetic testing relative to PGx has great potential, one hurdle that must be overcome for optimal implementation of personalized medicine is point-of-care testing. Here, we are not referring to whole-genome sequencing but rather specific testing for use in therapeutic decision making, such as testing an individual to identify his or her genotype relative to specific biomarkers (e.g., HLA, CYP2C19) related to drug therapy.

Technology is advancing in this realm as companies are working to develop point-of-care instruments for use in PGx-based therapy and dosing. A study utilizing rapid (one-hour) point-of-care genotyping showed its benefit in being able to initiate appropriate antiplatelet therapy in patients who underwent percutaneous coronary intervention for acute coronary syndrome or stable angina.[5] Patients were randomized to a PGx point-of-care testing group and prasugrel or to standard treatment with clopidogrel. All patients had platelet-activity testing. Based on this testing, all patients in the PGx testing/prasugrel group benefitted from the therapeutic choice, whereas 30% of patients in the standard treatment clopidogrel group did not benefit from treatment.[5] This was the first study to demonstrate the clinical applicability of point-of-care PGx testing. It is clear that the technology will continue to move to the bedside. Eventually, though, it is likely that whole-genome sequencing will replace this approach. At some point in the future when whole-genome sequencing is performed at the time of birth, the need for individual point-of-care testing, in the manner described, will cease. However, it will likely take years for this model to be implemented.

Data Storage and Presentation

Whole- or partial-genome sequencing results in the generation of extremely large quantities of data (e.g., terabytes to petabytes). Whereas the technology of sequencing used to be the rate-limiting step in moving genomics and PGx forward, today the bottleneck is related to data handling. For instance, as stated earlier, one direct-to-consumer company provides nearly 1,000,000 pieces of information to the individuals who utilize their services.

With technology poised to allow for the sequencing of millions of genomes in the near future, data storage, presentation, and interpretation will become critical if application of genomics, and PGx specifically, is to be realized on a large-scale basis. Bioinformatics—applying computer technology to gather, house, and analyze biologic data—will drive the utility of the data.[6,7] The clinical use of the data will only be made possible once data centers, healthcare facilities, and providers utilize electronic health records for communicating information. In the United States, the 2009 **Health Information Technology for Economic and Clinical Health (HITECH) Act** formed the Office of the National Coordinator for Health Information Technology. Through this office, dollars are being made available to design and implement an infrastructure to facilitate the use of electronic health records.[8] No matter how much data are generated, the realization of personalized medicine will not occur if the data cannot be communicated and interpreted appropriately.

Education

As noted above, the technology that has allowed more efficient sequencing of the human genome has resulted in an "information glut." The information being generated by genome sequencing has placed healthcare providers, health professions students, and the public in general on a steep learning curve.

Certainly, the field of PGx is not a core subject matter covered across all health professions curricula, although this is changing rapidly. In 2001, the National Coalition for Health Professional Education in Genetics (NCHPEG) published *Core Competencies in Genetics Essential for All Health-Care Professionals*.[9] Additionally, the 2001–2002 American Association of Colleges of Pharmacy Academic Affairs Committee recommended that PGx be included in colleges/schools of pharmacy curricula in recognition that genetics plays an inherent role in determining the pharmacokinetics and pharmacodynamics of drugs, resulting in a relationship between genetics and drug effects.[10]

A survey of colleges/schools of pharmacy relative to PGx education was performed in 2005, and a similar follow-up survey study was conducted in 2011.[11,12] Clearly, as **Table 11-1** indicates, colleges/schools of pharmacy have moved to integrate PGx into their curricula to a greater extent. Overall, 75% and 98% of colleges/schools of pharmacy included PGx in their curricula in 2005 and 2010, respectively.[11,12] Colleges/schools of pharmacy continue to increase PGx information in their curricula, and efforts have been made to provide comprehensive evidence-based educational content in PGx to colleges/schools that do not have their own content or want additional content to supplement their own.[13,14] This comprehensive offering includes a train-the-trainer program for faculty in colleges/schools of pharmacy as well as other healthcare education programs.[14] This component helps bring PGx/genomic expertise to institutions that do not have faculty with this background.[14]

Beyond the formal training of healthcare professions students, education of current practitioners is a necessity. A survey of more than 700 pharmacists revealed that more than 90% desired to learn more about **pharmacogenetics** and the utility of pharmacogenetic

Table 11-1

Pharmacogenetics and Pharmacogenomics at Colleges/Schools of Pharmacy

Question	2005 (n = 41) %	2010 (n = 75) %
Is pharmacogenetics/pharmacogenomics taught at your school?	78	92
Where does the subject reside in the PharmD curriculum?		
Standalone required didactic course.	9.8	21.7
Included as part of a required didactic course(s).	46.3	72.5
Elective didactic course.	2.4	34.8
What is the present state of pharmacogenomics instruction at most schools of pharmacy?		
Very Good	2.4	0
Good	9.8	2.7
Adequate	36.6	26.7
Poor	31.7	53.3
Not at all adequate	7.6	8
No response	11.9	9.3

Sources: Latif DA, McKay AB. Pharmacogenetics and pharmacogenomics instruction in colleges of pharmacy in the United States. *Am J Pharm Educ.* 2005;69(2):152–156; and Murphy JE, Green JS, Adams LA, et al. Pharmacogenomics in the curricula of colleges and schools of pharmacy in the United States. *Am J Pharm Educ.* 2010;74(1):1–10.

testing.[15] The case is similar, if not even more so, when considering other healthcare providers. A survey of over 10,000 physicians indicated that 10.3% felt they were adequately informed to utilize genetic testing, and only 29% had received formal training in PGx.[16] This underscores the current need for practitioners to be educated about the breadth of personalized medicine and speaks to the need of continuing education efforts in personalized medicine.[14,17–20] In fact, a review of education and training in PGx noted the "substantial coverage" of the subject in colleges of pharmacy as compared to schools of medicine, stating that "new learning models are needed to incentivize the training of physicians in genomics."[21]

Beyond healthcare providers and health professions students, the public in general must be educated on the subject of PGx. The National Human Genome Research Institute (NHGRI) provides public education opportunities related to genomics through outreach efforts aimed at high school students, special populations, and the public at large.[22] With respect to PGx, public education has been "called for" for over 10 years.[23,24] Much of the education will take place as healthcare providers utilize personalized medicine and explain the approach to their patients. Some institutions have included public education on PGx in their broader mission of education related to personalized medicine.[14] Clearly, once personalized medicine is adopted as a standard of care, education will be the job of all healthcare professionals.

Ethics and Discrimination

As the public in general and healthcare providers specifically encounter the growing world of medical applications of genetic information, ethical issues must be understood and addressed. The topics of ethical, legal, and social implications (ELSI) of genetic testing are broad and intricate and can be far reaching.

Patient autonomy is an inherent part of medical decision making. For example, the patient has the right to decide to receive a particular treatment, such as one for cancer, or the decision to undergo organ transplantation, among other independent decisions.[25] Oftentimes the decision is shared between the healthcare provider (or team) and the patient.[25] With genetic information, such as that provided by direct-to-consumer companies, patients have complete autonomy to share what information they choose. Certainly, there is a concern that individuals may not understand the potential consequences of sharing genetic information in that the information may be related to their sibling(s) and/or children; that is, related DNA between family members puts genetic information into a larger context. Autonomy is a key part of genetic information privacy; however, the general public likely needs to be educated to fully understand the results of whole- or partial-genome testing.

Privacy and confidentiality related to genetic information is not unlike that for other medical information, and it must be considered paramount in the provider–patient relationship. Certainly the **Health Insurance Portability and Accountability Act (HIPAA)** has provided a regulatory framework for privacy that allows appropriate disclosure of health information.[26]

Issues related to the ethics of genetic testing encompass the shared nature of DNA information, ownership of DNA data, inappropriate use of genetic testing, and the potential for discrimination, among other important topics.

With regard to discrimination, the **Genetic Information Nondiscrimination Act (GINA)** directly addresses discrimination by health insurers and employers relative to an individual's DNA that may impart risk of disease. The act, signed into federal law in 2008, prevents discrimination by health insurers and employers based on an individual's genetic information. However, discrimination by other entities, such as life insurers, lenders, and others is being addressed. For instance, in 2012 CalGINA, the California Genetic Information Nondiscrimination Act, went into effect.[27] This act extended nondiscrimination protection beyond just health insurers and employers.[27] It is likely that other individual states will consider broader-reaching genetic information nondiscrimination legislation.

Pharmacogenomics Resources

Numerous PGx resources are available for individuals to utilize that will provide greater depth and breadth in understanding the scientific basis for and application of genetic information/data.

PHARMGKB

PharmGKB, the "Pharmacogenomics Knowledgebase," is available online at www.pharmgkb.org. PharmGKB is an extensive database and resource that organizes, presents, and disseminates information and knowledge concerning genetic variation as it relates to drug response.[28] It includes annotations of relationships between genes, drugs, and disease that are supported by vetted literature. The resource provides researchers and clinicians with up-to-date information from reliable sources. Of particular interest to pharmacists and other clinicians, the site serves as a dissemination portal for pharmacogenomic-based drug dosing guidelines produced by the

Clinical Pharmacogenetics Implementation Consortium (CPIC).[29] The CPIC guidelines are a joint effort between PharmGKB and the Pharmacogenetics Research Network (PGRN) to aid clinicians in the clinical application of PGx. The CPIC guidelines also are published in the journal *Clinical Pharmacology and Therapeutics*. At this time, guidelines have been published for the gene–drug pairs thiopurine methyltransferase–thiopurines,[30] CYP2C19–clopidogrel,[31] CYP2C9–VKORC1–warfarin,[32] CYP2D6–codeine,[33] HLA-B-abacavir,[34] and SLCO1B1-simvastatin.[35] Additional guidelines to be published include DPYD–5-fluorouracil/capecitabine, HLA-B–carbamazepine, HLA-B–phenytoin, HLA-B–allopurinol, G6PD–rasburicase–Septra, UGT1A1–irinotecan, IL28B–pegintron, CYP2D6–CYP2C19–tricyclic antidepressants, and CYP2D6–selective serotonin reuptake inhibitors.[36] The PharmGKB project is supported by the National Institutes of Health/National Institute of General Medical Services and is managed by Stanford University.

DBSNP

The Single Nucleotide Polymorphism database (dbSNP) is a public-domain database of a diverse compilation of simple genetic polymorphisms. It is provided by the National Center for Biotechnology Information (NCBI) of the U.S. National Library of Medicine.[37] The dbSNP was designed mainly to support research across a wide range of technical areas, such as physical mapping of nucleotide sequences, including genes related to drug response variation; functional analysis of specific regions of genes that relate variation of a region to expression of a protein, such as a drug metabolizing enzyme (part of PGx); association studies of gene variation related to complex genetic traits; and evolutionary studies, where genome diversity is recognized. This database can be used to search for specific SNPs by utilizing dbSNP record identifiers, including reference SNP (refSNP) numbers. These numbers are unique and consistent identifiers of a given SNP.[38]

OTHER RESOURCES

Although not described in detail here, some other potentially useful resources can be found at the Pharmacogenomics Resources website (http://epi.grants.cancer.gov/pharm/gen-resources.html) of the National Cancer Institute (NCI).[39] This site is a portal to collaborative opportunities, consortia, networks, databases, knowledge-synthesis resources, presentations and reports, and toolkits.[39] Additionally, the Genetics/Genomics Competency Center G2C2 (www.g-2-c-2.org) houses genomic information and is a portal to vetted resource information for nurses, physician assistants, genetic counselors, and, in the near future, pharmacists.[40]

Chapter Summary

Advances in technology have made DNA sequencing a reality, and it will move personalized medicine to the forefront of patient care. However, most individuals will be on a steep learning curve, which will slow the implementation of personalized medicine. Individuals will work to become expert at interpretation of data, while communication of the information will require a framework of privacy and nondiscrimination. To facilitate the understanding of PGx information, a number of resources have been developed, including important drug-dosing guidelines that support clinical decision making.

Review Questions

1. As technology advances relative to genome sequencing, the goal is to have a sequencing method that is:
   a. $10,000.
   b. $10.
   c. $1,000 or less.
   d. $5,000.

2. _____ is the discipline of applying computer technology to gather, house, and analyze biological data.
   a. Pharmacogenetics
   b. Bioinformatics
   c. Pharmacogenomics
   d. Pharmacokinetics
   e. Bio-analysis

3. Which of the following is the federal law that is concerned with the privacy and portability of healthcare information?
   a. HITECH
   b. PGx
   c. FDA
   d. GINA
   e. HIPAA

4. A 2012 survey of pharmacists identified that greater than
_____ of those surveyed desired to learn more about pharmacogenetics and the utility of pharmacogenetic testing.
   a. 90%
   b. 70%
   c. 50%
   d. 20%
   e. 10%

5. The Genetic Information Nondiscrimination Act (GINA; 2008)
prevents _____ from discriminating based on an individual's genetic information.
   a. lenders and borrowers
   b. lawyers and law enforcement
   c. life insurers and actuaries
   d. health insurers and employers

6. CPIC guidelines are available through which of the following?
   a. dbSNP
   b. C-Path
   c. PharmGKB
   d. RS#
   e. RefSNP

7. In general, resources for pharmacogenomics information
include or will include which of the following?
   a. dbSNP
   b. PharmGKB
   c. G2C2
   d. a and c only
   e. a, b, and c

References

1. Sanger F, Nicklen S, Coulson AR. DNA sequencing with chain-terminating inhibitors. *Proc Natl Acad Sci.*1977;74(12):5463–5467.
2. DNA sequencing costs. Available at: www.genome.gov/sequencingcosts. Accessed April 24, 2012.
3. Wade N. Cost of decoding a genome is lowered. *New York Times*, August 2010.
4. Clarke J, Wu HC, Jayasinghe L, et al. Continuous base identification for single-molecule nanopore DNA sequencing. *Nat Nabotech.* 2009;4:265–270.

5. Roberts JD, Wells GA, Le May MR, et al. Point-of-care genetic testing for personalisation of antiplatelet treatment (RAPID GENE): A prospective, randomised, proof-of-concept trial. *Lancet.* 2012;5;379(9827):1705–1711.

6. Koboldt DC, Ding L, Mardis ER, Wilson RK. Challenges of sequencing human genomes. *Brief Bioinform.* 2010;11(5):484–498.

7. National Center for Biotechnology Information. Just the facts: A basic introduction to the science underlying NCBI Resources: BIOINFORMATICS. Available at: www.ncbi.nlm.nih.gov/About/primer/bioinformatics.html. Accessed April 24, 2012.

8. Office of the National Coordinator for Health Information Technology. Available at: http://healthit.hhs.gov/portal/server.pt/community/healthit _hhs_gov__home/1204. Accessed April 26, 2012.

9. National Coalition for Health Professional Education in Genetics. *Core competencies in genetics essential for all health-care professionals.* Lutherville, MD: Author; 2001.

10. Johnson JA, Bootman JL, Evans WE, et al. Pharmacogenomics: A scientific revolution in pharmaceutical sciences and pharmacy practice. Report of the 2001–2002 Academic Affairs Committee. *Am J Pharm Educ.* 2002;66(9):12S–156S.

11. Latif DA, McKay AB. Pharmacogenetics and pharmacogenomics instruction in colleges of pharmacy in the United States. *Am J Pharm Educ.* 2005;69(2):152–156;

12. Murphy JE, Green JS, Adams LA, et al. Pharmacogenomics in the curricula of colleges and schools of pharmacy in the United States. *Am J Pharm Educ.* 2010;74(1):1–10.

13. Springer JA, Iannotti NV, Kane MD, Haynes K, Sprague JE. Pharmacogenomics training using an instructional software system. *J Pharm Educ.* 2011;75(2):32.

14. Kuo GM, Ma1 JD, Lee KC, et al. University of California San Diego Pharmacogenomics Education Program (PharmGenEd™): Bridging the gap between science and practice. *Pharmacogenomics.* 2011;12(2):149–153.

15. Roederer MW, Riper MV, Valgus J, Knafl G, McLeod H. Knowledge, attitudes and education of pharmacists regarding pharmacogenetic testing. *Personal Med.* 2012;9:19–27.

16. Stanek EJ, Sanders CL, Johansen Taber KA, et al. Adoption of pharmacogenomic testing by US physicians: Results of a nationwide survey. *Clin Pharmacol Ther.* 2012;91(3):450–458.

17. Likovich M, Derr A, Kane MD, Kisor DF, Sprague JE. Personalized medicine and the future of pharmacy practice. *Pharmacy Times.* 2010 (April). Available at: https://secure.pharmacytimes.com/lessons/201004-01.asp. Accessed March 27, 2012.

18. Kisor DF, Munro C, Loudermilk E. Pharmacogenomics and the most commonly prescribed drugs of 2011. *Pharmacy Times.* 2012 (in press).

19. Kane JM. Clinical insights into pharmacogenetics and schizophrenia. CME Institute. Available at: www.cmeinstitute.com/series_home.asp?SID=78. Accessed April 12, 2012.

20. Ventura M, Desko L, Gathers K, Overy A, Kisor DF. Genetic variation in a cytochrome P450 enzyme and the effects on clopidogrel bioactivation and metabolism. *Pharmacy Wellness Rev.* 2011;2(1):8–13.

21. Lesko LJ, Johnson JA. Academia at the crossroads: Education and training in pharmacogenomics. *Personal Med.* 2012;9(5):497–506.

22. National Human Genome Research Institute. Community outreach and public education. Available at: www.genome.gov/10001279. Accessed April 25, 2012.

23. Grant SFA. Pharmacogenetics and pharmacogenomics: tailored drug therapy for the 21st century. *Trends Pharmacol Sci.* 2001;22(1):3–4.

24. Frueh FW, Goodsaid F, Rudman A, Huang S-M, Lesko LJ. The need for education in pharmacogenomics: a regulatory perspective. *Pharmacogenomics J.* 2005;5:218–220.

25. Drake RE, Cimpean D, Torrey WC. Shared decision making in mental health: Prospects for personalized medicine. *Dialogues Clin Neurosci.* 2009;11(4):455–463.

26. U.S. Department of Health and Human Services. Understanding health information privacy. Available at: www.hhs.gov/ocr/privacy/hipaa/understanding/index.html. Accessed April 26, 2012.

27. California Genetic Information Nondiscrimination Act. Available at: www.leginfo.ca.gov/ pub/11-12/bill/sen/sb_0551-0600/sb_559_bill_20110906_chaptered.pdf. Accessed May 1, 2012.

28. PharmGKB. The Pharmacogenomics Knowledgebase. Available at: www.pharmgkb.org. Accessed July 23, 2012.

29. PharmGKB. Clinical Pharmacogenetics Implementation Consortium. Available at: www.pharmgkb.org/page/cpic. Accessed July 22, 2012.

30. Relling MV, Gardner EE, Sandborn WJ, et al. Clinical Pharmacogenetics Implementation Consortium guidelines for thiopurine methyltransferase genotype and thiopurine dosing. *Clin Pharmacol Ther.* 2011;89(3):387–391.

31. Scott SA, Sangkuhl K, Gardner EE, et al. Clinical Pharmacogenetics Implementation Consortium guidelines for cytochrome P450-2C19 (CYP2C19) genotype and clopidogrel therapy. *Clin Pharmacol Ther.* 2011;90(2):328–332.

32. Johnson JA, Gong L, Whirl-Carrillo M, et al. Clinical Pharmacogenetics Implementation Consortium Guidelines for CYP2C9 and VKORC1 genotypes and warfarin dosing. *Clin Pharmacol Ther.* 2011;90(4):625–629.

33. Crews KR, Gaedigk A, Dunnenberger HM, et al. Clinical Pharmacogenetics Implementation Consortium (CPIC) guidelines for codeine therapy in the context of cytochrome P450 2D6 (CYP2D6) genotype. *Clin Pharmacol Ther.* 2012;91(2):321–326.

34. Martin MA, Klein TE, Dong BJ, Pirmohamed M, Haas DW, Kroetz DL. Clinical Pharmacogenetics Implementation Consortium guidelines for HLA-B genotype and abacavir dosing. *Clin Pharmacol Ther.* 2012;91(4):734–738.

35. Wilke RA, Ramsey LB, Johnson SG, et al. The Clinical Pharmacogenomics Implementation Consortium: CPIC guideline for SLCO1B1 and simvastatin-induced myopathy. *Clin Pharmacol Ther.* 2012;92(1):112–117.

36. PharmGKB. Gene–drug pairs. Available at: www.pharmgkb.org/page/cpicGeneDrugPairs. Accessed July 29, 2012.

37. dbSNP. The Single Nucleotide Polymorphism Database (dbSNP) of Nucleotide Sequence Variation. Available at: www.ncbi.nlm.nih.gov/SNP/index.html. Accessed July 29, 2012.

38. Kitts A, Sherry S. The Single Nucleotide Polymorphism Database (dbSNP) of nucleotide sequence variation. Available at: www.ncbi.nlm.nih.gov/books/NBK21088. Accessed July 12, 2012.

39. National Cancer Institute. Pharmacogenomic resources. Available at: http://epi.grants.cancer.gov/pharm/gen-resources.html. Accessed July 19, 2012.

40. G2C2 Genetics/Genomics Competency Center. Available at: www.g-2-c-2.org. Accessed August 9, 2012.

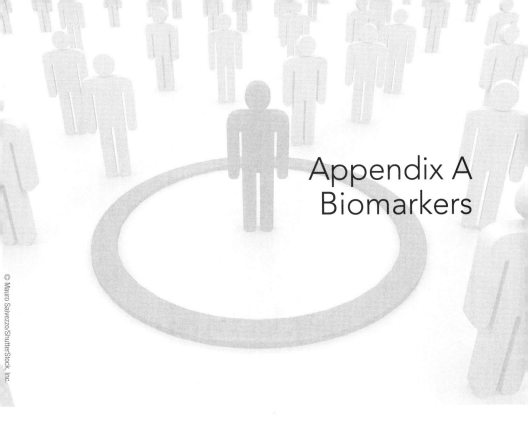

Appendix A
Biomarkers

In the context of this text, a biomarker is defined as a protein generated by genes that is related to a drug enzyme (e.g., CYP2D6), a drug transporter (e.g., P-glycoprotein), or a drug target (e.g., β_2-adrenergic receptors) as well as other cellular components that can be analyzed and predictive of pharmacokinetics and pharmacodynamics related to drug response.

The Food and Drug Administration (FDA) provides a "Table of Valid Biomarkers" that presents approved drugs with pharmacogenomic information in specified sections of the package labeling. **Tables A-1** and **A-2** are two adaptations of the table, with information provided through August 16, 2012. The first adaptation, Table A-1, presents the information listed by biomarker and distinguishes the biomarker as related to pharmacokinetics (PK) and/or pharmacodynamics (PD). The second adaptation, Table A-2, presents the information listed by therapeutic area. The FDA table is regularly updated, and the student is encouraged to visit the FDA website for the most up-to-date information. The table can be found at www.fda.gov/drugs/scienceresearch/researchareas/pharmacogenetics/ucm083378.htm.

Table A-1

Drugs Listed by Biomarker Related to Pharmacokinetics and/or Pharmacodynamics

PK/PD	Biomarker	Drug	Therapeutic Area	Package Label Section(s)
PD	ALK[a]	Crizotinib	Oncology	Indications and Usage, Warnings and Precautions, Adverse Reactions, Clinical Pharmacology, Clinical Studies
PD	ApoE2[b]	Pravastatin	Metabolic and Endocrinology	Clinical Studies, Use in Specific Populations
PD	BRAF[c]	Vemurafenib	Oncology	Indications and Usage, Warnings and Precautions, Clinical Pharmacology, Clinical Studies, Patient Counseling Information
PD	CCR5[d]	Maraviroc	Antivirals	Indications and Usage, Warnings and Precautions, Clinical Pharmacology, Clinical Studies, Patient Counseling Information
PD	CD20[e] antigen	Tositumomab	Oncology	Indications and Usage, Clinical Pharmacology
PD	CD25[f]	Denileukin diftitox	Oncology	Indications and Usage, Warnings and Precautions, Clinical Studies
PD	CD30[g]	Brentuximab vedotin	Oncology	Indications and Usage, Description, Clinical Pharmacology
PD	CFTR[h] (G551D)	Ivacaftor	Pulmonary	Indications and Usage, Adverse Reactions, Use in Specific Populations, Clinical Pharmacology, Clinical Studies
PD	Chromosome 5q[i]	Lenalidomide	Hematology	Boxed Warning, Indications and Usage, Clinical Studies, Patient Counseling
PD	C-Kit[j]	Imatinib	Oncology	Indications and Usage, Dosage and Administration Clinical Pharmacology, Clinical Studies
PK	CYP1A2[k]	Dexlansoprazole	Gastroenterology	Clinical Pharmacology
PK	CYP2C19[l]	Carisoprodol	Musculoskeletal	Clinical Pharmacology, Special Populations
PK	CYP2C19[l]	Citalopram	Psychiatry	Drug Interactions, Warnings
PK	CYP2C19[l]	Clobazam	Neurology	Clinical Pharmacology, Dosage and Administration, Use in Specific Populations
PK	CYP2C19[l]	Clopidogrel	Cardiovascular	Boxed Warning, Dosage and Administration, Warnings and Precautions, Drug Interactions, Clinical Pharmacology

PK/PD	Biomarker	Drug	Therapeutic Area	Package Label Section(s)
PK	CYP2C19[l]	Dexlansoprazole	Gastroenterology	Clinical Pharmacology, Drug Interactions
PK	CYP2C19[l]	Diazepam	Psychiatry	Drug Interactions, Clinical Pharmacology
PK	CYP2C19[l]	Drospirenone and ethinyl estradiol	Reproductive	Precautions, Drug Interactions
PK	CYP2C19[l]	Esomeprazole	Gastroenterology	Drug Interactions, Clinical Pharmacology
PK	CYP2C19[l]	Omeprazole	Gastroenterology	Dosage and Administration, Warnings and Precautions, Drug Interactions
PK	CYP2C19[l]	Pantoprazole	Gastroenterology	Clinical Pharmacology, Drug Interactions, Special Populations
PK	CYP2C19[l]	Prasugrel	Cardiovascular	Use in Specific Populations, Clinical Pharmacology, Clinical Studies
PK	CYP2C19[l]	Rabeprazole	Gastroenterology	Drug Interactions, Clinical Pharmacology
PK	CYP2C19[l]	Ticagrelor	Cardiovascular	Clinical Studies
PK	CYP2C19[l]	Voriconazole	Antifungals	Clinical Pharmacology, Drug Interactions
PK	CYP2C9[m]	Celecoxib	Analgesics	Dosage and Administration, Drug Interactions, Use in Specific Populations, Clinical Pharmacology
PK	CYP2C9[m]	Flurbiprofen	Rheumatology	Clinical Pharmacology, Special Populations
PK	CYP2C9[m]	Warfarin	Hematology	Dosage and Administration, Precautions, Clinical Pharmacology
PK	CYP2D6[n]	Aripiprazole	Psychiatry	Clinical Pharmacology, Dosage and Administration
PK	CYP2D6[n]	Atomoxetine	Psychiatry	Dosage and Administration, Warnings and Precautions, Drug Interactions, Clinical Pharmacology
PK	CYP2D6[n]	Carvedilol	Cardiovascular	Drug Interactions, Clinical Pharmacology
PK	CYP2D6[n]	Cevimeline	Dermatology and Dental	Drug Interactions
PK	CYP2D6[n]	Chlordiazepoxide and amitriptyline	Psychiatry	Precautions
PK	CYP2D6[n]	Citalopram	Psychiatry	Drug Interactions
PK	CYP2D6[n]	Clomipramine	Psychiatry	Drug Interactions
PK	CYP2D6[n]	Clozapine	Psychiatry	Drug Interactions, Clinical Pharmacology
PK	CYP2D6[n]	Codeine	Analgesics	Warnings and Precautions, Use in Specific Populations, Clinical Pharmacology
PK	CYP2D6[n]	Desipramine	Psychiatry	Drug Interactions

(continues)

Table A-1
(continued)

PK/PD	Biomarker	Drug	Therapeutic Area	Package Label Section(s)
PK	CYP2D6[n]	Dextromethorphan and quinidine	Neurology	Clinical Pharmacology, Warnings and Precautions
PK	CYP2D6[n]	Doxepin	Psychiatry	Precautions
PK	CYP2D6[n]	Fluoxetine	Psychiatry	Warnings, Precautions, Clinical Pharmacology
PK	CYP2D6[n]	Fluoxetine and olanzapine	Psychiatry	Drug Interactions, Clinical Pharmacology
PK	CYP2D6[n]	Fluvoxamine	Psychiatry	Drug Interactions
PK	CYP2D6[n]	Galantamine	Neurology	Special Populations
PK	CYP2D6[n]	Iloperidone	Psychiatry	Clinical Pharmacology, Dosage and Administration, Drug Interactions, Specific Populations, Warnings and Precautions
PK	CYP2D6[n]	Imipramine	Psychiatry	Drug Interactions
PK	CYP2D6[n]	Metoprolol	Cardiovascular	Precautions, Clinical Pharmacology
PK	CYP2D6[n]	Modafinil	Psychiatry	Drug Interactions
PK	CYP2D6[n]	Nefazodone	Psychiatry	Drug Interactions
PK	CYP2D6[n]	Nortriptyline	Psychiatry	Drug Interactions
PK	CYP2D6[n]	Paroxetine	Psychiatry	Clinical Pharmacology, Drug Interactions
PK	CYP2D6[n]	Perphenazine	Psychiatry	Clinical Pharmacology, Drug Interactions
PK	CYP2D6[n]	Pimozide	Psychiatry	Warnings, Precautions, Contraindications, Dosage and Administration
PK	CYP2D6[n]	Propafenone	Cardiovascular	Clinical Pharmacology
PK	CYP2D6[n]	Propranolol	Cardiovascular	Precautions, Drug Interactions, Clinical Pharmacology
PK	CYP2D6[n]	Protriptyline	Psychiatry	Precautions
PK	CYP2D6[n]	Quinidine	Antiarrhythmics	Precautions
PK	CYP2D6[n]	Risperidone	Psychiatry	Drug Interactions, Clinical Pharmacology
PK	CYP2D6[n]	Terbinafine	Antifungals	Drug Interactions

PK/PD	Biomarker	Drug	Therapeutic Area	Package Label Section(s)
PK	CYP2D6[n]	Tetrabenazine	Neurology	Dosage and Administration, Warnings, Clinical Pharmacology
PK	CYP2D6[n]	Thioridazine	Psychiatry	Precautions, Warnings, Contraindications
PK	CYP2D6[n]	Tolterodine	Reproductive and Urologic	Clinical Pharmacology, Drug Interactions, Warnings and Precautions
PK	CYP2D6[n]	Tramadol and acetaminophen	Analgesics	Clinical Pharmacology
PK	CYP2D6[n]	Trimipramine	Psychiatry	Drug Interactions
PK	CYP2D6[n]	Venlafaxine	Psychiatry	Drug Interactions
PK	DPD[o]	Capecitabine	Oncology	Contraindications, Precautions, Patient Information
PK	DPD[o]	Fluorouracil	Dermatology and Dental	Contraindications, Warnings
PD	EGFR[p]	Cetuximab	Oncology	Indications and Usage, Warnings and Precautions, Description, Clinical Pharmacology, Clinical Studies
PD	EGFR[p]	Erlotinib	Oncology	Clinical Pharmacology
PD	EGFR[p]	Gefitinib	Oncology	Clinical Pharmacology
PD	EGFR[p]	Panitumumab	Oncology	Indications and Usage, Warnings and Precautions, Clinical Pharmacology, Clinical Studies
PD	ER &/ PgR[r] receptor[q]	Exemestane	Oncology	Indications and Usage, Dosage and Administration, Clinical Studies, Clinical Pharmacology
PD	ER[q] &/ PgR[r] receptor	Letrozole	Oncology	Indications and Usage, Adverse Reactions, Clinical Studies, Clinical Pharmacology
PD	ER[q] receptor	Fulvestrant	Oncology	Indications and Usage, Patient Counseling Information
PD	ER[q] receptor	Tamoxifen	Oncology	Indications and Usage, Precautions, Medication Guide
PD	FIP1L1-PDGFRα[s]	Imatinib	Oncology	Indications and Usage, Dosage and Administration, Clinical Studies
PD	G6PD[t]	Chloroquine	Anti-infectives	Precautions
PD	G6PD[t]	Dapsone	Dermatology and Dental	Indications and Usage, Precautions, Adverse Reactions, Patient Counseling Information
PD	G6PD[t]	Rasburicase	Oncology	Boxed Warning, Contraindications
PD	Her2/neu[u]	Everolimus	Oncology	Indications and Usage, Boxed Warning, Adverse Reactions, Use in Specific Populations, Clinical Pharmacology, Clinical Studies

(continues)

Table A-1
(continued)

PK/PD	Biomarker	Drug	Therapeutic Area	Package Label Section(s)
PD	Her2/neu[u]	Lapatinib	Oncology	Indications and Usage, Clinical Pharmacology, Patient Counseling Information
PD	Her2/neu[u]	Pertuzumab	Oncology	Indications and Usage, Warnings and Precautions, Adverse Reactions, Clinical Studies, Clinical Pharmacology
PD	Her2/neu[u]	Trastuzumab	Oncology	Indications and Usage, Precautions, Clinical Pharmacology
PD	HLA-B*1502[v]	Carbamazepine	Neurology	Boxed Warning, Warnings and Precautions
PD	HLA-B*1502[v]	Phenytoin	Neurology	Warnings
PD	HLA-B*5701[w]	Abacavir	Antivirals	Boxed Warning, Contraindications, Warnings and Precautions, Patient Counseling Information
PD	IL28B[x]	Boceprevir	Antivirals	Clinical Pharmacology
PD	IL28B[x]	Peginterferon alfa-2b	Antivirals	Clinical Pharmacology
PD	IL28B[x]	Telaprevir	Antivirals	Clinical Pharmacology
PD	KRAS[y]	Cetuximab	Oncology	Indications and Usage, Dosage and Administration, Warnings and Precautions, Adverse Reactions, Clinical Pharmacology, Clinical Studies
PD	KRAS[y]	Panitumumab	Oncology	Indications and Usage, Clinical Pharmacology, Clinical Studies
PD	LDLR[z]	Atorvastatin	Metabolic and Endocrinology	Indications and Usage, Dosage and Administration, Warnings and Precautions, Clinical Pharmacology, Clinical Studies
PK	NAT1; NAT2[aa]	Isosorbide and hydralazine	Cardiovascular	Clinical Pharmacology
PK	NAT1; NAT2[aa]	Rifampin, isoniazid, and pyrazinamide	Anti-infectives	Adverse Reactions, Clinical Pharmacology
PD	PDGFR[bb]	Imatinib	Oncology	Indications and Usage, Dosage and Administration, Clinical Studies
PD	Ph chromosome[cc]	Busulfan	Oncology	Clinical Studies
PD	Ph chromosome[cc]	Imatinib	Oncology	Indications and Usage, Dosage and Administration, Clinical Pharmacology, Clinical Studies
PD	Ph chromosome[cc]	Nilotinib	Oncology	Indications and Usage, Patient Counseling Information

PK/PD	Biomarker	Drug	Therapeutic Area	Package Label Section(s)
PD	PML/RARα[dd]	Arsenic trioxide	Oncology	Boxed Warning, Clinical Pharmacology, Indications and Usage, Warnings
PD	PML/RARα[dd]	Tretinoin	Dermatology and Dental	Boxed Warning, Dosage and Administration, Precautions
PD	Rh genotype[ee]	Clomiphene	Reproductive and Urologic	Precautions
PK	TPMT[ff]	Azathioprine	Rheumatology	Dosage and Administration, Warnings and Precautions, Drug Interactions, Adverse Reactions, Clinical Pharmacology
PK	TPMT[ff]	Cisplatin	Oncology	Clinical Pharmacology, Warnings, Precautions
PK	TPMT[ff]	Mercaptopurine	Oncology	Dosage and Administration, Contraindications, Precautions, Adverse Reactions, Clinical Pharmacology
PK	TPMT[ff]	Thioguanine	Oncology	Dosage and Administration, Precautions, Warnings
PD	UCD (NAGS; CPS; ASS; OTC; ASL; ARG)[gg]	Sodium phenylacetate and sodium benzoate	Gastroenterology	Indications and Usage, Description, Clinical Pharmacology
PD	UCD (NAGS; CPS; ASS; OTC; ASL; ARG)[gg]	Sodium phenylbutyrate	Gastroenterology	Indications and Usage, Dosage and Administration, Nutritional Management
PD	UCD (NAGS; CPS; ASS; OTC; ASL; ARG)[gg]	Valproic acid	Psychiatry	Contraindications, Precautions, Adverse Reactions
PK	UGT1A1[hh]	Indacaterol	Pulmonary	Clinical Pharmacology
PK	UGT1A1[hh]	Irinotecan	Oncology	Dosage and Administration, Warnings, Clinical Pharmacology
PK	UGT1A1[hh]	Nilotinib	Oncology	Warnings and Precautions, Clinical Pharmacology
PD	VKORC1[ii]	Warfarin	Hematology	Dosage and Administration, Precautions, Clinical Pharmacology

[a] Anaplastic lymphoma kinase; [b] apolipoprotein (allele) E2; [c] v-raf murine sarcoma viral oncogene homolog B1; [d] chemokine receptor 5; [e] B-cell surface protein; [f] IL-2 receptor alpha chain; [g] alymphocyte activation antigen; [h] cystic fibrosis transmembrane conductance regulator gene; [i] chromosome 5 (relative to deletion syndrome); [j] a receptor tyrosine kinase protein; [k] cytochrome P-450 enzyme family 1 subfamily A individual member 2; [l] cytochrome P-450 enzyme family 2 subfamily C individual member 19; [m] cytochrome P-450 enzyme family 2 subfamily C individual member 9; [n] cytochrome P-450 enzyme family 2 subfamily D individual member 6; [o] dihydropyrimidine dehydrogenase; [p] epidermal growth factor receptor; [q] estrogen receptor; [r] progesterone receptor; [s] cleavage and polyadenylation specificity factor and platelet-derived growth factor receptor alpha; [t] glucose-6-phosphate dehydrogenase; [u] human epidermal growth factor receptor 2; [v] human leukocyte antigen (major histocompatibility complex, class I, B) of a specific allele family (15); [w] human leukocyte antigen (major histocompatibility complex, class I, B) of a specific allele family (57); [x] interluekin 28 B; [y] kirsten RNA associated rat sarcoma 2 virus gene; [z] low density lipoprotein receptor; [aa] n-acetyltransferase; [bb] platelet derived growth factor receptor; [cc] Philadelphia chromosome; [dd] promyelocytic leukemia/retinoic acid receptor; [ee] rhesus factor; [ff] thiopurine methyltransferase; [gg] urea cycle disorder; [hh] uridine diphosphate glucuronosyltransferase 1A1; [ii] vitamin K epoxide reductase complex subunit 1.

Table A-2

Drugs Listed by Therapeutic Area

Therapeutic Area	Drug	Biomarker	Package Label Section(s)
Analgesics	Celecoxib	CYP2C9	Dosage and Administration, Drug Interactions, Use in Specific Populations, Clinical Pharmacology
Analgesics	Codeine	CYP2D6	Warnings and Precautions, Use in Specific Populations, Clinical Pharmacology
Analgesics	Tramadol and acetaminophen	CYP2D6	Clinical Pharmacology
Antiarrhythmics	Quinidine	CYP2D6	Precautions
Antifungals	Voriconazole	CYP2C19[l]	Clinical Pharmacology, Drug Interactions
Antifungals	Terbinafine	CYP2D6	Drug Interactions
Anti-infectives	Chloroquine	G6PD	Precautions
Anti-infectives	Rifampin, isoniazid, and pyrazinamide	NAT1; NAT2	Adverse Reactions, Clinical Pharmacology
Antivirals	Maraviroc	CCR5[d]	Indications and Usage, Warnings and Precautions, Clinical Pharmacology, Clinical Studies, Patient Counseling Information
Antivirals	Abacavir	HLA-B*5701	Boxed Warning, Contraindications, Warnings and Precautions, Patient Counseling Information
Antivirals	Boceprevir	IL28B	Clinical Pharmacology
Antivirals	Peginterferon alfa-2b	IL28B	Clinical Pharmacology
Antivirals	Telaprevir	IL28B	Clinical Pharmacology
Cardiovascular	Clopidogrel	CYP2C19[l]	Boxed Warning, Dosage and Administration, Warnings and Precautions, Drug Interactions, Clinical Pharmacology
Cardiovascular	Prasugrel	CYP2C19[l]	Use in Specific Populations, Clinical Pharmacology, Clinical Studies
Cardiovascular	Ticagrelor	CYP2C19[l]	Clinical Studies
Cardiovascular	Carvedilol	CYP2D6	Drug Interactions, Clinical Pharmacology
Cardiovascular	Metoprolol	CYP2D6	Precautions, Clinical Pharmacology
Cardiovascular	Propafenone	CYP2D6	Clinical Pharmacology

Therapeutic Area	Drug	Biomarker	Package Label Section(s)
Cardiovascular	Propranolol	CYP2D6	Precautions, Drug Interactions, Clinical Pharmacology
Cardiovascular	Isosorbide and hydralazine	NAT1; NAT2	Clinical Pharmacology
Dermatology and Dental	Cevimeline	CYP2D6	Drug Interactions
Dermatology and Dental	Fluorouracil	DPD	Contraindications, Warnings
Dermatology and Dental	Dapsone	G6PD	Indications and Usage, Precautions, Adverse Reactions, Patient Counseling Information
Dermatology and Dental	Tretinoin	PML/RARα	Boxed Warning, Dosage and Administration, Precautions
Gastroenterology	Dexlansoprazole	CYP1A2[k]	Clinical Pharmacology
Gastroenterology	Dexlansoprazole	CYP2C19[l]	Clinical Pharmacology, Drug Interactions
Gastroenterology	Esomeprazole	CYP2C19[l]	Drug Interactions, Clinical Pharmacology
Gastroenterology	Omeprazole	CYP2C19[l]	Dosage and Administration, Warnings and Precautions, Drug Interactions
Gastroenterology	Pantoprazole	CYP2C19[l]	Clinical Pharmacology, Drug Interactions, Special Populations
Gastroenterology	Rabeprazole	CYP2C19[l]	Drug Interactions, Clinical Pharmacology
Gastroenterology	Sodium phenylacetate and sodium benzoate	UCD (NAGS; CPS; ASS; OTC; ASL; ARG)	Indications and Usage, Description, Clinical Pharmacology
Gastroenterology	Sodium phenylbutyrate	UCD (NAGS; CPS; ASS; OTC; ASL; ARG)	Indications and Usage, Dosage and Administration, Nutritional Management
Hematology	Lenalidomide	Chromosome 5q[i]	Boxed Warning, Indications and Usage, Clinical Studies, Patient Counseling
Hematology	Warfarin	CYP2C9	Dosage and Administration, Precautions, Clinical Pharmacology
Hematology	Warfarin	VKORC1	Dosage and Administration, Precautions, Clinical Pharmacology
Metabolic and Endocrinology	Pravastatin	ApoE2[b]	Clinical Studies, Use in Specific Populations
Metabolic and Endocrinology	Atorvastatin	LDL receptor	Indications and Usage, Dosage and Administration, Warnings and Precautions, Clinical Pharmacology, Clinical Studies

(continues)

Table A-2
(continued)

Therapeutic Area	Drug	Biomarker	Package Label Section(s)
Musculoskeletal	Carisoprodol	CYP2C19[l]	Clinical Pharmacology, Special Populations
Neurology	Clobazam	CYP2C19[l]	Clinical Pharmacology, Dosage and Administration, Use in Specific Populations
Neurology	Dextromethorphan and quinidine	CYP2D6	Clinical Pharmacology, Warnings and Precautions
Neurology	Galantamine	CYP2D6	Special Populations
Neurology	Tetrabenazine	CYP2D6	Dosage and Administration, Warnings, Clinical Pharmacology
Neurology	Carbamazepine	HLA-B*1502	Boxed Warning, Warnings and Precautions
Neurology	Phenytoin	HLA-B*1502	Warnings
Oncology	Crizotinib	ALK[a]	Indications and Usage, Warnings and Precautions, Adverse Reactions, Clinical Pharmacology, Clinical Studies
Oncology	Vemurafenib	BRAF[c]	Indications and Usage, Warnings and Precautions, Clinical Pharmacology, Clinical Studies, Patient Counseling Information
Oncology	Tositumomab	CD20[e] antigen	Indications and Usage, Clinical Pharmacology
Oncology	Denileukin diftitox	CD25[f]	Indications and Usage, Warnings and Precautions, Clinical Studies
Oncology	Brentuximab vedotin	CD30[g]	Indications and Usage, Description, Clinical Pharmacology
Oncology	Imatinib	C-Kit[j]	Indications and Usage, Dosage and Administration Clinical Pharmacology, Clinical Studies
Oncology	Capecitabine	DPD	Contraindications, Precautions, Patient Information
Oncology	Cetuximab	EGFR	Indications and Usage, Warnings and Precautions, Description, Clinical Pharmacology, Clinical Studies
Oncology	Erlotinib	EGFR	Clinical Pharmacology
Oncology	Gefitinib	EGFR	Clinical Pharmacology
Oncology	Panitumumab	EGFR	Indications and Usage, Warnings and Precautions, Clinical Pharmacology, Clinical Studies

Therapeutic Area	Drug	Biomarker	Package Label Section(s)
Oncology	Exemestane	ER &/ PgR receptor	Indications and Usage, Dosage and Administration, Clinical Studies, Clinical Pharmacology
Oncology	Letrozole	ER &/ PgR receptor	Indications and Usage, Adverse Reactions, Clinical Studies, Clinical Pharmacology
Oncology	Fulvestrant	ER receptor	Indications and Usage, Patient Counseling Information
Oncology	Tamoxifen	ER receptor	Indications and Usage, Precautions, Medication Guide
Oncology	Imatinib	FIP1L1-PDGFRα	Indications and Usage, Dosage and Administration, Clinical Studies
Oncology	Rasburicase	G6PD	Boxed Warning, Contraindications
Oncology	Everolimus	Her2/neu	Indications and Usage, Boxed Warning, Adverse Reactions, Use in Specific Populations, Clinical Pharmacology, Clinical Studies
Oncology	Lapatinib	Her2/neu	Indications and Usage, Clinical Pharmacology, Patient Counseling Information
Oncology	Pertuzumab	Her2/neu	Indications and Usage, Warnings and Precautions, Adverse Reactions, Clinical Studies, Clinical Pharmacology
Oncology	Trastuzumab	Her2/neu	Indications and Usage, Precautions, Clinical Pharmacology
Oncology	Cetuximab	KRAS	Indications and Usage, Dosage and Administration, Warnings and Precautions, Adverse Reactions, Clinical Pharmacology, Clinical Studies
Oncology	Panitumumab	KRAS	Indications and Usage, Clinical Pharmacology, Clinical Studies
Oncology	Imatinib	PDGFR	Indications and Usage, Dosage and Administration, Clincal Studies
Oncology	Busulfan	Ph chromosome	Clinical Studies
Oncology	Dasatinib	Ph chromosome	Indications and Usage, Clinical Studies, Patient Counseling Information
Oncology	Imatinib	Ph chromosome	Indications and Usage, Dosage and Administration, Clinical Pharmacology, Clinical Studies
Oncology	Nilotinib	Ph chromosome	Indications and Usage, Patient Counseling Information

(continues)

Table A-2
(continued)

Therapeutic Area	Drug	Biomarker	Package Label Section(s)
Oncology	Arsenic trioxide	PML/RARα	Boxed Warning, Clinical Pharmacology, Indications and Usage, Warnings
Oncology	Cisplatin	TPMT	Clinical Pharmacology, Warnings, Precautions
Oncology	Mercaptopurine	TPMT	Dosage and Administration, Contraindications, Precautions, Adverse Reactions, Clinical Pharmacology
Oncology	Thioguanine	TPMT	Dosage and Administration, Precautions, Warnings
Oncology	Irinotecan	UGT1A1	Dosage and Administration, Warnings, Clinical Pharmacology
Oncology	Nilotinib	UGT1A1	Warnings and Precautions, Clinical Pharmacology
Psychiatry	Citalopram	CYP2C19l	Drug Interactions, Warnings
Psychiatry	Diazepam	CYP2C19	Drug Interactions, Clinical Pharmacology
Psychiatry	Aripiprazole	CYP2D6	Clinical Pharmacology, Dosage and Administration
Psychiatry	Atomoxetine	CYP2D6	Dosage and Administration, Warnings and Precautions, Drug Interactions, Clinical Pharmacology
Psychiatry	Chlordiazepoxide and amitriptyline	CYP2D6	Precautions
Psychiatry	Citalopram	CYP2D6	Drug Interactions
Psychiatry	Clomipramine	CYP2D6	Drug Interactions
Psychiatry	Clozapine	CYP2D6	Drug Interactions, Clinical Pharmacology
Psychiatry	Desipramine	CYP2D6	Drug Interactions
Psychiatry	Doxepin	CYP2D6	Precautions
Psychiatry	Fluoxetine	CYP2D6	Warnings, Precautions, Clinical Pharmacology
Psychiatry	Fluoxetine and olanzapine	CYP2D6	Drug Interactions, Clinical Pharmacology
Psychiatry	Fluvoxamine	CYP2D6	Drug Interactions
Psychiatry	Iloperidone	CYP2D6	Clinical Pharmacology, Dosage and Administration, Drug Interactions, Specific Populations, Warnings and Precautions
Psychiatry	Imipramine	CYP2D6	Drug Interactions

Therapeutic Area	Drug	Biomarker	Package Label Section(s)
Psychiatry	Modafinil	CYP2D6	Drug Interactions
Psychiatry	Nefazodone	CYP2D6	Drug Interactions
Psychiatry	Nortriptyline	CYP2D6	Drug Interactions
Psychiatry	Paroxetine	CYP2D6	Clinical Pharmacology, Drug Interactions
Psychiatry	Perphenazine	CYP2D6	Clinical Pharmacology, Drug Interactions
Psychiatry	Pimozide	CYP2D6	Warnings, Precautions, Contraindications, Dosage and Administration
Psychiatry	Protriptyline	CYP2D6	Precautions
Psychiatry	Risperidone	CYP2D6	Drug Interactions, Clinical Pharmacology
Psychiatry	Thioridazine	CYP2D6	Precautions, Warnings, Contraindications
Psychiatry	Trimipramine	CYP2D6	Drug Interactions
Psychiatry	Venlafaxine	CYP2D6	Drug Interactions
Psychiatry	Valproic Acid	UCD (NAGS; CPS; ASS; OTC; ASL; ARG)	Contraindications, Precautions, Adverse Reactions
Pulmonary	Ivacaftor	CFTR[h] (G551D)	Indications and Usage, Adverse Reactions, Use in Specific Populations, Clinical Pharmacology, Clinical Studies
Pulmonary	Indacaterol	UGT1A1	Clinical Pharmacology
Reproductive	Drospirenone and ethinyl estradiol	CYP2C19[l]	Precautions, Drug Interactions
Reproductive and Urologic	Tolterodine	CYP2D6	Clinical Pharmacology, Drug Interactions, Warnings and Precautions
Reproductive and Urologic	Clomiphene	Rh genotype	Precautions
Rheumatology	Flurbiprofen	CYP2C9	Clinical Pharmacology, Special Populations
Rheumatology	Azathioprine	TPMT	Dosage and Administration, Warnings and Precautions, Drug Interactions, Adverse Reactions, Clinical Pharmacology

[a] Anaplastic lymphoma kinase; [b] apolipoprotein (allele) E2; [c] v-raf murine sarcoma viral oncogene homolog B1; [d] chemokine receptor 5; [e] B-cell surface protein; [f] IL-2 receptor alpha chain; [g] a lymphocyte activation antigen; [h] cystic fibrosis transmembrane conductance regulator gene; [i] chromosome 5 (relative to deletion syndrome); [j] a receptor tyrosine kinase protein; [k] cytochrome P-450 enzyme family 1 subfamily A individual member 2; [l] cytochrome P-450 enzyme family 2 subfamily C individual member 19; [m] cytochrome P-450 enzyme family 2 subfamily C individual member 9; [n] cytochrome P-450 enzyme family 2 subfamily D individual member 6; [o] dihydropyrimidine dehydrogenase; [p] epidermal growth factor receptor; [q] estrogen receptor; [r] progesterone receptor; [s] cleavage and polyadenylation specificity factor and platelet-derived growth factor receptor alpha; [t] glucose-6-phosphate dehydrogenase; [u] human epidermal growth factor receptor 2; [v] human leukocyte antigen (major histocompatibility complex, class I, B) of a specific allele family (15); [w] human leukocyte antigen (major histocompatibility complex, class I, B) of a specific allele family (57); [x] interleukin 28 B; [y] kirsten RNA associated rat sarcoma 2 virus gene; [z] low density lipoprotein receptor; [aa] n-acetyltransferase; [bb] platelet derived growth factor receptor; [cc] Philadelphia chromosome; [dd] promyelocytic leukemia/retinoic acid receptor; [ee] rhesus factor; [ff] thiopurine methyltransferase; [gg] urea cycle disorder; [hh] uridine diphosphate glucuronosyltransferase 1A1; [ii] vitamin K epoxide reductase complex subunit 1.

Appendix B
Pharmacogenomics and the Most Commonly Prescribed Drugs

Pharmacogenomics may be viewed as a new discipline by many pharmacists. However, pharmacogenomic information is found in the package labels of some of the most commonly prescribed medications. When considering the list of the top 200 drugs as presented by *Pharmacy Times*, by total prescriptions in 2011, 17 included pharmacogenomic information in their package labeling, including the 5th and 7th most commonly prescribed drugs (see **Table B-1**). In 2011, in total, more than 362 million prescriptions were filled for these 17 drugs. This number is certain to increase dramatically as personalized medicine progresses.

Table B-1

Therapeutic Areas with Examples of Drugs for Which There Is Pharmacogenomic Information in the Package Label

Therapeutic Area: Drug Example (Top 200 Rank 2011)[a,b]	Biomarker	Package Label Section(s)
Metabolic and endocrinology—atorvastatin (5)	LDLR[c]	Indications and Usage, Dosage and Administration, Warnings and Precautions, Clinical Pharmacology, Clinical Studies
Cardiovascular—clopidogrel (7)	CYP2C19[d]	Boxed Warning, Dosage and Administration, Warnings and Precautions, Drug Interactions, Clinical Pharmacology
Gastroenterology—omeprazole (21)	CYP2C19[d]	Dosage and Administration, Warnings and Precautions, Drug Interactions
Analgesics—tramadol (25)	CYP2D6[e]	Clinical Pharmacology
Hematology—warfarin (35)	CYP2C9[f]/VKORC1[g]	Dosage and Administration, Precautions, Clinical Pharmacology
Cardiovascular—pravastatin (38)	ApoE2[h]	Clinical Studies, Use in Specific Populations
Cardiovascular—metoprolol (40)	CYP2D6[e]	Precautions, Clinical Pharmacology
Psychiatry—fluoxetine (65)	CYP2D6[e]	Warnings, Precautions, Clinical Pharmacology
Psychiatry—citalopram (67)	CYP2C19[d]/CYP2D6[e]	Drug Interactions
Psychiatry—venlafaxine (75)	CYP2D6[e]	Drug Interactions
Cardiovascular—carvedilol (86)	CYP2D6[e]	Drug Interactions, Clinical Pharmacology
Psychiatry—diazepam (105)	CYP2C19[d]	Drug Interactions, Clinical Pharmacology
Psychiatry—amitriptyline (120)	CYP2D6[e]	Precautions
Psychiatry—paroxetine (143)	CYP2D6[e]	Clinical Pharmacology, Drug Interactions
Musculoskeletal—carisoprodol (148)	CYP2C19[d]	Clinical Pharmacology, Special Populations
Psychiatry—risperidone (157)	CYP2D6[e]	Drug Interactions, Clinical Pharmacology
Gastroenterology—pantoprazole (193)	CYP2C19[d]	Clinical Pharmacology, Drug Interactions, Special Populations

[a] Highest ranking; [b] all manufacturers and dosage forms; [c] low density lipoprotein receptor; [d] cytochrome P-450 enzyme family 2 subfamily C individual member 19; [e] cytochrome P-450 enzyme family 2 subfamily D individual member 6; [f] cytochrome P-450 enzyme family 2 subfamily C individual member 9; [g] vitamin K epoxide reductase complex subunit 1; [h] apolipoprotein (allele) E2.

Source: Pharmacy Times. 2011 Top 200 drugs. Available at: www.pharmacytimes.com/publications/ issue/2012/July2012 /Top-200-Drugs-of-2011. Accessed August 23, 2012.

Appendix C
Personalized
Medicine and Me

The case presented here describes how an individual examined his risk of disease and drug response information using actual genome data provided by a direct-to-consumer genetic testing company. "Personalized Medicine and Me" provides an example of how genomic information could be provided for all individuals in the future. Currently, in the clinical setting individual genetic tests (e.g., CYP2C19) are ordered to support specific decision making relative to a patient's drug therapy or other clinical question. It is likely that this approach will be replaced by whole-genome sequencing, likely at the time of birth. In the future, the genetic-testing results will be stored securely and will be available for query throughout an individual's life.

This example provides real data obtained from a saliva sample provided by the given individual. Although not based on whole-genome sequencing, the genetic testing provided more than 950,000 SNPs that were available for query, depending on the individual's particular needs. Here, the individual makes the assumption that the genetic testing was performed using a valid analytical procedure.

The Process

The first step is ordering a testing kit. Certainly, this is not how the process will work at the time of birth, when testing (in the future) will likely be performed; however, this is the current process the individual completed. The kit was ordered online from the genetic-testing company. The company offered choices for different "levels" of service (e.g., monthly updates related to new genetic discoveries). The product was identified, online registration was completed, and payment was made by credit card. In approximately one week, the testing kit arrived via standard U.S. Postal Service delivery. The kit contained specific instructions, which the individual read completely before obtaining the sample. Following the directions, the saliva sample was provided. It took about 5 minutes and involved spitting into a tube to obtain the required volume. The plastic tube containing the saliva was then capped. The tube's cap had a compartment that contained a DNA stabilization buffer, and upon securing the cap the buffer automatically mixed with the saliva. The tube was then inverted a number of times to ensure thorough mixing of the saliva and buffer. At this point the "shipping cap" was placed on the tube, replacing the cap that contained the buffer. The tube was placed in the provided ziplock "biohazard-bag" and placed into a preaddressed return container. An email was sent at the time the results were ready for viewing. After agreeing to online consent questions, the results were made available via the online portal.

Disease Risk Data

The results included the following information relative to the individual's genetic-based increased risk for disease (see **Table C-1**). We present only the information with adequate scientific and clinical research support.

Table C-1			
Diseases for Which the Individual Has an Increased Risk, Based on Genetic Testing			
Disease	Individual's Risk[a] (%)	Population Average Risk (%)	Ratio: Individual/ Population
Prostate cancer	26.7	17.8	1.50
Venous thromboembolism	17.9	12.3	1.45
Rheumatoid arthritis	2.9	2.4	1.20
Ulcerative colitis	1.0	0.8	1.25

[a] Relative risk.

Table C-2		
Single Nucleotide Polymorphisms (SNPs) Related to Prostate Cancer		
SNP	**Genotype**	**Comment**
rs1447295	CC	Average risk
rs6983267	GT	1.2 × the average risk
rs1859962	GT	Average risk
rs4430796	AA	1.38 × the average risk
rs16901979	CC	Average risk

To understand how this information may be used, the results from the genetic testing of the individual's saliva provided the information shown in **Table C-2** relative to prostate cancer risk.

The first four SNPs listed in Table C-2 were provided in a summary section of results. The four SNPs, plus a fifth SNP, rs16901979, were individually related to risk of prostate cancer and collectively, with a family history, had a cumulative association with prostate cancer.[1] The fifth SNP, rs16901979, was not provided in the summary results; however, the genetic-testing company provided the "raw SNP data," which included 960,613 SNPs. The SNP database was queried (search term "rs16901979"), and the search returned the following information:

RefSNP ID: rs16901979   Chromosome: 8   Genotype: CC

The CC genotype, in the context of Table C-2, provides information on rs16901979.

This individual has two SNPs with genotypes that impart an increased risk of prostate cancer; however, this is a relative risk, and it does not mean that the individual will definitely develop this cancer. This is the individual's attempt at understanding the data, and the interpretation may not be accurate. It is presented here as an example. Most importantly, the individual has undergone appropriate screening with a physical examination and lab work, showing a prostate specific antigen value of 1.18 ng/mL, with less than 4 ng/mL being considered normal. The individual will continue to follow standard screening with the guidance of his physician.

Drug Response Data

The summary data provided the following information regarding two drugs for which the response was different from "normal." **Table C-3** shows the results that are related to the term "response."

The prodrug clopidogrel is metabolized to its active form via CYP2C19. Additionally, relative to altered metabolism and activation

Table C-3	
Drug Response Data from the Direct-to-Consumer Genetic Testing Company	
Name	**Status**
Clopidogrel (Plavix) Efficacy	Reduced
Warfarin (Coumadin) Sensitivity	Increased

of clopidogrel, the CYP2C19*2 allele is the most common loss-of-function variant. The polymorphism is noted as c.681G>A, with the reference SNP number rs4244285. Searching the individual's data, the following is noted:

RefSNP ID: rs4244285 Chromosome: 10 Genotype: AG

Therefore, this individual is heterozygous with a CYP2C19*1/*2 genotype and would be considered an intermediate metabolizer. If the individual requires antiplatelet therapy, it is recommended that he receive prasugrel or another antiplatelet drug instead of clopidogrel.[2]

With regard to warfarin, pharmacokinetic and pharmacodynamic variability is introduced by genetic variation. Here, CYP2C9 is related to warfarin metabolism, whereas the genomic biomarker vitamin K epoxide reductase complex subunit 1 (VKORC1) is the target enzyme for the drug.

The most common reduced-function CYP2C9 variants are the *2 and *3 forms, seen in white, Asian, and black individuals at frequencies of 0.13, 0, 0.03 and 0.07, 0.04, and 0.02, respectively.[3] The CYP2C9*2 variant has the reference SNP number rs1799853, and the CYP2C9*3 variant is rs1057910. Individuals with the *2 or *3 variants have decreased metabolism of warfarin and require reduced doses of the drug. Searching the individual's data, the following is noted:

RefSNP ID: rs1799853 Chromosome 10 Position: 96702047
Genotype: CC

RefSNP ID: rs1057910 Chromosome 10 Position: 96741053
Genotype: AA

The cytosine at position 96702047 and the adenine at position 96741053 on each of the two number 10 chromosomes impart "normal" extensive metabolism of warfarin (i.e., these are not variant alleles), and the individual is a CYP2C9*1/*1 (wild-type) individual.

The warfarin target, VKORC1, can be present in a variant form, with rs9923231 (−1639G>A, also known as 1173C>T) imparting warfarin sensitivity due to decreased VKORC1 expression. Essentially, in this case less warfarin is needed to inhibit VKORC1.

Again, searching the individual's genetic data, the following information is retrieved:

RefSNP ID: rs9923231 Chromosome 16 Position: 31107689
Genotype: TT

Therefore, this individual would require a lower maintenance dose of warfarin, not because of decreased metabolism of the drug, but rather due to increased "sensitivity" as VKORC1 expression is decreased.

This case of an individual being able to query his SNP data is an example of what may occur in the future with whole-genome sequencing data. Once the data are obtained, the storage and retrieval of the needed information will be of utmost importance; that is, keeping the data secure, but accessible in appropriate situations, such as determining the correct drug or dose of a drug when there is a relationship between genetics and drug response.

Note that this example refers to data from a direct-to-consumer (DTC) company. The U.S. General Accounting Office (GAO) has determined that different DTC companies provide different, if not contrary, disease risk results and caution that interpretation of the data could be difficult and that results from some companies may be misleading. Additionally, deceptive advertising practices have been noted for a number of companies.[4]

The individual in the above case provided samples to the company on two different occasions, and the results were identical. The individual believed the raw data to be accurate. With respect to the genetic data related to the drugs, the individual confirmed the CYP2C19*2 variant using a research laboratory approach. The key to the future use of genetic data will be the availability of valid genomic data provided by reputable laboratories. Consumers should be cautioned when utilizing DTC genetic testing.

References

1.   Zheng SL, Sun J, Wiklund F, et al. Cumulative association of five genetic variants with prostate cancer. N Engl J Med. 2008;358:910–919.
2.   Scott SA, Sangkuhl K, Gardner EE, et al. Clinical Pharmacogenetics Implementation Consortium guidelines for cytochrome P450-2C19 (CYP2C19) genotype and clopidogrel therapy. Clin Pharmacol Ther. 2011;90(2):328–332.
3.   Johnson JA, Gong L, Whirl-Carrillo M, et al. Clinical Pharmacogenetics Implementation Consortium (CPIC) Guidelines for CYP2C9 and VKORC1 Genotypes and Warfarin Dosing—ONLINE SUPPLEMENT. Available at: www.pharmgkb.org/drug/PA451906. Accessed August 22, 2012.
4.   U.S. Government General Accountability Office (GAO). Direct-to-consumer genetic tests: Misleading test results are further complicated by deceptive marketing and other questionable practices. Available at: www.gao.gov/products/GAO-10-847T. Accessed August 21, 2012.

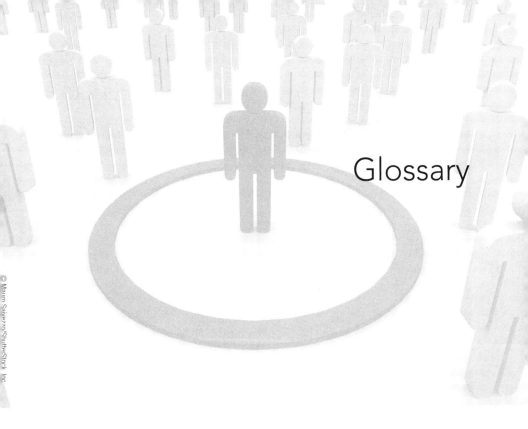

Glossary

absorption rate constant (k_a; time^{-1}) The rate constant representing the first-order absorption of drug from an extravascular site (e.g., gastrointestinal tract).

affinity The strength of the reversible interaction between a drug and a drug target (receptor).

agonist An endogenous or exogenous ligand that activates a drug target to induce a response.

allele Alternate sequences or versions of the same gene inherited from each parent.

antagonist An endogenous or exogenous ligand that attenuates another endogenous or exogenous ligand from activating a drug target to induce a response.

area under the curve (AUC; amt/vol · time) A measure of drug exposure as the integrated area under the plasma drug concentration versus time curve from time zero to infinity.

bioavailability (F) The rate and extent of drug absorption; the fraction of the dose reaching systemic circulation unchanged.

biomarker (genomic) A measurable DNA and/or RNA characteristic that is an indicator of normal biologic processes, pathogenic processes, and/or response to therapeutic or other interventions.

$C_{ss,ave}$ **(amt/vol)** The average steady-state drug concentration.

clearance (CL; vol/time) The volume of biologic fluid from which drug is removed per unit time.

codon Three adjacent nucleotide bases that ultimately encodes a specific amino acid.

CYP; CYP450 The cytochrome P450 oxidative metabolic enzyme superfamily.

dissociation constant (K_D) The ratio of free drug (D) and receptor (R) concentration to drug-receptor [DR] concentration. Used to determine the affinity of an agonist.

drug resistance The inability of a drug to produce a pharmacodynamic response at a standard dose.

drug target Endogenous binding sites for drugs. Drug targets can include receptors, enzymes, and membrane transporters.

EC_{50} The half-maximal (50%) effective concentration of a drug producing a specific response.

efficacy The effect (E) elicited by a drug (D) and the concentration of drug–receptor complex [DR].

efflux transporter A protein that moves drug out of cells/tissues.

elimination rate constant (k_e; time^{-1}) The rate constant representing the first-order elimination of drug from a one-compartment model.

exon A nucleotide sequence that codes information for protein synthesis.

extensive metabolizer (EM) An individual with two "normal-function" alleles relative to a drug metabolizing enzyme.

gene Regions of the genome (DNA) that contain the instructions to make proteins.

Genetic Information Nondiscrimination Act (GINA) Act by Congress that prohibits discrimination of an individual by health insurers and employers based on the individual's genetic information.

genome The entire DNA of an organism.

genotype The specific set of alleles inherited at a locus on a given gene.

haplotype A series of polymorphisms that are inherited together.

Health Insurance Portability and Accountability Act (HIPAA) Act by Congress that allows individuals to keep their health insurance when they change or lose their job; decreases healthcare fraud and abuse; requires medical information confidentiality; and regulates industry standards related to medical billing and other processes.

Health Information Technology for Economic and Clinical Health Act (HITECH) Part of the 2009 Recovery and Reinvestment Act mandating the use of electronic health records, primarily by physicians and hospitals.

heterozygous Possessing two different alleles for the same trait.

histone A protein around which DNA coils to form chromatin, thus "packaging" the DNA.

homozygous Possessing identical alleles for the same trait.

IC_{50} The antagonist concentration eliciting a 50% reduction in response (inhibition).

indel Insertion or deletion of DNA either as single nucleotides or spanning regions of DNA involving many nucleotides.

influx (uptake) transporter A protein that moves drug into cells/tissues.

intermediate metabolizer (IM) In general, an individual with one "loss-of-function" allele and one "normal-function" allele relative to a drug metabolizing enzyme.

intron A nucleotide sequence in DNA that does not code information for protein synthesis and is removed before translation of messenger RNA.

K_i Affinity of an antagonist drug for a receptor.

ligand Endogenous or exogenous agent that binds to a drug target.

loading dose (D_L; amt) The initial dose of a drug; administered with the intent of producing a near steady-state average concentration.

maximum concentration (C_{max}; amt/vol) Highest concentration of drug in biologic fluid following drug administration during a dosing interval.

minimum concentration (C_{min}; amt/vol) Lowest concentration of drug in biologic fluid following drug administration during a dosing interval. Typically occurring immediately before a subsequent dose.

monogenic trait Characteristics derived from a single gene.

multigenic trait Characteristics derived from multiple genes.

mutation A change in DNA sequence between individuals.

nucleotide One of the structural components, or building blocks, of DNA, including adenine (A), cytosine (C), guanine (G), and thymine (T), and of RNA, including adenine (A), cytosine (C), guanine (G), and (U) uracil.

personalized medicine The use of patient-specific information and biomarkers to make more informed choices regarding the optimal therapeutic treatment regimen for a given patient.

pharmacodynamics (PD) The relationship between drug exposure and pharmacologic response.

pharmacogenetics (PGt) The study of a gene involved in response to a drug.

pharmacogenomics (PGx) The study of many genes, in some cases the entire genome, involved in response to a drug.

pharmacokinetics (PK) The relationship of time and drug absorption, distribution, metabolism, and excretion.

phase 1 metabolism Drug metabolizing processes involving oxidation, reduction, or hydrolysis.

phase 2 metabolism Conjugative drug metabolizing processes.

phenotype An individual's expression of a physical trait or physiologic function due to genetic makeup and environmental and other factors.

polymorphism A mutation in DNA in a given population that may be observed at greater than 1% frequency.

poor metabolizer (PM) An individual with two "reduced-function" or "loss-of-function" alleles relative to a drug metabolizing enzyme.

potency The dependence of the pharmacologic effect(s) of the drug on the drug concentration.

prodrug A drug that requires conversion to an active form.

reference sequence number (refSNP; rs#) A unique and consistent identifier of a given single nucleotide polymorphism (SNP).

serotonin reuptake transporter (SERT) A transport protein that regulates the amounts of serotonin in the synaptic cleft.

single nucleotide polymorphism (SNP) A variant DNA sequence in which a single nucleotide has been replaced by another base.

tau (τ; time) The dosing interval.

T_{max} (time) The time of occurrence of the maximum concentration of drug.

topoisomerase A class of enzymes that alter the supercoiling of double-stranded DNA.

ultrarapid metabolizer (UM) An individual with two "gain-of-function" alleles (e.g., overexpression of a metabolic enzyme). In general, having increased metabolizing enzyme activity relative to an extensive metabolizer.

volume of distribution (V, Vd, V_1, Vss; vol) A proportionality constant relating the amount of drug in the body with the drug concentration.

wild-type The typical or normally occurring genotype of an organism.

xenobiotics Substances (often drugs) introduced into the body but not produced by it.

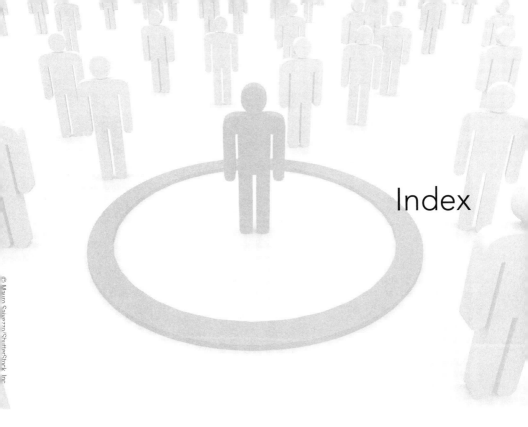

Index

Note: For drug names beginning with a numeral (e.g., 6-mercaptopurine), the numeral is ignored in alphabetization. Figures are indicated by f following the page number and tables by t.